# Nurses of All Nations

**A History of the International Council of Nurses, 1899-1999**

# Nurses of All Nations

## A History of the International Council of Nurses, 1899-1999

EDITORS

**Barbara L. Brush, PhD, RN**

Assistant Professor
School of Nursing
Boston College
Chestnut Hill, Massachusetts

**Joan E. Lynaugh, PhD, RN, FAAN**

Emeritus Professor
Center for the Study of the History of Nursing
School of Nursing
University of Pennsylvania
Philadelphia, Pennsylvania

---

**Geertje Boschma, PhD**

Assistant Professor
University of Alberta
Faculty of Nursing
Edmonton, Alberta, Canada

**Meryn Stuart, PhD**

Associate Professor
School of Nursing
University of Ottawa
Ottawa, Ontario, Canada

**Anne Marie Rafferty, PhD**

Director
Centre for Policy in Nursing Research
London School of Hygiene and Topical Medicine
London, England

**Nancy J. Tomes, PhD**

Professor
State University of New York at Stony Brook
Stony Brook, New York

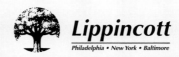

*Lippincott*

Philadelphia • New York • Baltimore

*Vice President & Publisher:* Donna L. Hilton, RN, BSN
*Coordinating Editorial Assistant:* Bridget Blatteau
*Associate Managing Editor:* Barbara Ryalls
*Senior Production Manager:* Helen Ewan
*Production Coordinator:* Patricia McCloskey
*Design Coordinator:* Doug Smock
*Indexer:* Michael Ferreira

9    8    7    6    5    4    3    2    1

Library of Congress Cataloging-in-Publication Data

Nurses of all nations : a history of the International Council of
Nurses, 1899–1999 / editors, Barbara L. Brush . . . [et al.].
    p. cm.
Includes bibliographical references and index.
ISBN 0-7817-1904-6 (alk. paper)
    1. Nursing—Societies—History 20th century. 2. International
Council of Nurses. I. Brush, Barbara L.
RT1.N758 1999
610.73′06′01—dc21                                    98-37564
                                                          CIP

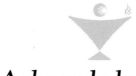

# Acknowledgments

This book is the culmination of more than a decade of planning, consulting, research, and writing. In 1987, Constance Holleran, then Executive Director of the International Council of Nurses, broached the idea of doing a new history marking the occasion of ICN's 100th anniversary. For 3 years she persisted, with support from the ICN Board of Directors and historical consultation from Ellen D. Baer, until the project was finally launched by the six of us in 1990. In a decision vital to the book's historical validity, ICN granted us free access to all historic documents and assured our academic control over the resulting book. We benefited from repeated and generous consultation with Ellen Baer, Karen Buhler-Wilkerson, Marianne Tallberg, and, of course, Connie Holleran. Former and present ICN officers patiently responded to our requests for information and clarification, as did staff and officers of the many national nursing associations we contacted. Special thanks for helping in myriad ways go to Judith Oulton, Fadwa Affara, Mireille Kingma, Taka Oguisso, Sarojini Patel, and Nancy Vatre in ICN's Geneva office. Past and present staff at the Center for the Study of the History of Nursing at the University of Pennsylvania, especially Carla Castillo, Elizabeth Weiss, and Margo Szabunia, enabled every facet of the project. We appreciate the enthusiastic confidence of Vice President and Publisher Donna Hilton of Lippincott Williams & Wilkins. And finally, we thank our families, friends, and colleagues who shared with, supported, and listened to us through the many years of discussion, research, and writing leading to this day.

# Contents

# T H R E E

## Seeking Stability in the Midst of Change .................... 71

*Meryn Stuart, with Geertje Boschma*

# F O U R

## From Chaos to Transformation ............................... 111

*Joan E. Lynaugh*

# F I V E
## New Missions, New Meanings ................................. 149
*Barbara L. Brush*

# S I X

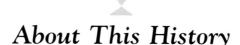

# About This History

JOAN E. LYNAUGH
AND BARBARA L. BRUSH
*for the ICN History Collective*

## Introduction

We find the roots of today's International Council of Nurses (ICN) in women's suffrage, abolition, missionary work, and social reform. Ethel Bedford Fenwick, Lavinia Dock, Agnes Karll, and the other founders of the ICN conceived of and believed in the link between women's rights and professional nursing. One hundred years ago, at the turn of this century, they began to build their new organization around that concept. The novel idea of self government by women through nurse-led national association proved popular and enduring. A steadily growing number of nurses from England and her colonies, from the United States, Canada, Germany, the Netherlands, and from Scandinavia ultimately chose to band together in the ICN during those early years. The strategy of state registration for nurses, the ideal of nursing as a higher vocation, and declaiming nurses as model women citizens captured their imagination and allegiance. Anxious to establish universal standards for nursing practice and confident of their western cultural superiority, the ICN nurses encouraged each other to form stronger national associations.

During their second decade of development, however, the advent of World War I, followed by turmoil in Russia and elsewhere, interrupted their plans and undermined their efforts. Throughout the 1920s, the ICN pulled itself back together and through the efforts of a small band of strong leaders struggled to emerge as an influential professional organization. After the war, demand for better public health and rebuilding of hospitals and health services, especially in Europe, created an opportunity for the ICN to provide leadership. With the International Red Cross, ICN helped set standards for new nursing schools and organizations. Chronic financial problems restrained the growth of the organization, but new members from China, Palestine, Brazil, and the Philippines attested to its more diverse international composition. Just as it was gaining stability, however, World War II broke out and once again external events threatened to dissolve the federation.

As was true of all of nursing, the ICN became caught up in and ultimately transformed by the worldwide destruction and political realignments of World War II. During the 1950s, the Anglo-European character of the organization began to change with the introduction of many new members from Africa, Asia, and South America. The ICN implemented a new, more global agenda, including the incorporation of many previously colonized countries as influential members. The organization became a stronger participant in postwar internationalism. However, political barriers erected during the Cold War inhibited the influence of the ICN in eastern Europe, Russia, and China. And economic, racial, religious, and gender issues continued to complicate the professional development of nursing in many countries. Nevertheless, the ICN defined nursing's work worldwide and claimed the right to speak for nursing in an ever wider sphere of influence.

The 1970s and 1980s became a period of rapid growth in the number of nurses represented by the ICN. Moreover, it faced issues ranging from the apartheid policies of South Africa's nursing association and torture of political prisoners in Chile, to more mundane redefinition of qualifications for membership. Tensions between international standards and preserving important national prerogatives kept the ICN Board and committee meetings lively and full of controversy. The ICN forged closer links with the World Health Organization and took an active part in efforts to improve the delivery of primary health care to people around the world. At the same time, the ICN took positions supporting the rights of nurses to fair employment and freedom from exploitation. By 1985 there were 97 countries federated within the ICN, representing 1,056,066 members. The ICN offered support and advice on issues such as the shortage of nurses and relations with physicians and other health workers in many countries.

As the first and most enduring professional organization founded by women, the ICN history speaks to women and men everywhere who aspire to direct their own affairs and fate. Founded 100 years ago to guide the professional development of nursing, the International Council of Nurses today is a federation of 120 member nurses' associations representing more than 1.5 million nurses from diverse backgrounds and settings. Now based in Geneva, Switzerland, its present-day mission is to provide leadership and assistance in resolving present and future health care needs.

## Themes and Approaches

As we researched and discussed the documents of the International Council, we came to share five perspectives on its 100-year story that we trace throughout the book. These five perspectives are the subtly changing self image of the ICN, its responses to issues of race, class, and gender, the meaning attached to nursing and profession, nursing diplomacy and organizational survival, and personal friendships and travel.

# Self Image

From the beginning, the women who founded and sustained the ICN consciously sought to create a shared identity and image. They struggled to find common ground when political, economic, or military events threatened them and their solidarity. Over time, the foremost task of the ICN was to find, and find again, as circumstances changed, an organizational identity with meaning and utility for nurses from different cultures, political and religious belief systems, economic structures, and organizational experiences.

# Race, Class and Gender

This is a history that, because of the nature of the ICN mission and federation, encompasses aspects of colonialism, the western missionary movement, the women's movements of the 19th and 20th centuries, the "hot wars" (especially World Wars I and II) and the "Cold War," the trade union movement, decolonization, social justice, and human rights. It is not comfortable to read accounts of Western nurses superimposing their ways on colonial populations or other peoples, either through missionary work or through the state. Nursing, so intimate in its work, faithfully mirrors both the unattractive and the uplifting aspects of the human experience. We find white domination, racial and religious segregation, and class exploitation. We also find what American ICN founder Lavinia Dock called the "four lions" lying in the path of nurse solidarity: male dominance, religious prejudice, class prejudice, and the century-long debate between trade unionism and professionalism.

# Meaning of Nursing and Profession

For nearly 100 years, the two tasks of establishing educational standards and defining the nature of nursing remained significant to the ICN reason for being. British founder Ethel Bedford Fenwick and American Lavinia Dock believed that recognition of the trained and licensed nurse was both an end in itself and a means to social justice for women. Their commitment to better nursing education and a distinct, recognized definition of nursing was absolute. Later ICN leaders struggled to develop the idea of nursing distinctiveness using both scientific grounds and political argument, as well as by building power-sharing coalitions with other interested groups. Over and over again, the ICN leaders developed universally accepted standards and definitions for nursing and spread these formulations around the world by any means they could.

## Nursing Diplomacy

The ICN has no country but it has endured as a kind of "nursing state" for 100 years. The uniqueness of that historical fact intrigued and often perplexed us as historians. How the ICN created and maintained its place in the world over time is what we came to call "nursing diplomacy." In the beginning, people like Ethel Gordon Fenwick and Lavinia Dock simply and defiantly declared that they were in charge of the future of nursing. Later, during the 1920s, the organization "stayed alive" by very active negotiation and compromise on the part of ICN Presidents Sophie Mannerheim and Nina Gage and Executive Secretary Christianne Reimann. And then, as the ICN emerged from World War II, it sought out and found a role for itself in the community of international organizations.

The relationship between nurses, the state, and the profession is a truly fascinating perspective on the history of the ICN. From the beginning, ICN leaders assumed they must achieve state protection and recognition of their work in all the nations of the world. They could not seek recognition from universities, which were becoming the western world's means of labeling professional distinctiveness. They had no significant access to universities because most nurses were women and because nursing was considered neither "learned" nor a profession. Nor did they wish to use the trade union model to protect their craft. So, a significant task of the ICN became finding a way to get each nation state to acknowledge the profession and accredit the individual professional nurse.

## Friendship

And finally, we found that one simple but vital ingredient in the "glue" that created and sustained the ICN was the friendship, collegial support, and enthusiasm for one another found in generation after generation of nurses. Nurses seemingly have always loved to travel and discover others like and unlike themselves around the world. The loyalty nurses displayed toward their profession in the abstract and to each other in the personal sense seemed often the only way to explain how they could repeatedly transcend the discord and violence so characteristic of the 20th century.

## Writing the History of the ICN

Other historians studying the history of the ICN might well interpret it from other vantage points. But these five themes, organizational image, race, class and gender, meaning of nursing and profession, nursing diplomacy, and friendship and travel, helped us place successive generations of nurses in the ICN in the perspective of their own time and context.

This is a history of the events and people at the center of the ICN federation, and institutional history. It is not a history of all, or even some of the national nursing organizations. There are, however, many fine such histories which are listed in an appendix to this book.

We enjoyed full access to all ICN archives and materials. Trips to the ICN archives in Geneva, Switzerland and to other collections in Europe, Canada, and the USA, searches of the professional literature, a review of 20th-century historical scholarship, a search for and survey of national histories of nursing, interviews of contemporary leaders, and a series of lengthy meetings among the six historians laid the groundwork for our individual research and helped us frame this history. The documentary evidence held by the ICN, as well as the other materials of its leaders, found scattered in various archives in Europe and the USA, is quite extensive. Various other entities, especially the International Red Cross and the Rockefeller Foundation, maintain important and relevant collections. New and older histories of nursing, public health, and medicine contain material related to ICN events or biographical information on ICN actors. We also obtained valuable consultation from international historians working on specific aspects of this history who generously shared both insights and materials. We divided the research and writing into six segments, with each chapter specifically authored by one or two of the group. Barbara Brush and Joan Lynaugh edited the book.

The ICN has a rich historiography that served, we argue, to create and sustain its place in the world. For instance, many readers are familiar with Adelaide Nutting and Lavinia Dock's four-volume history completed in 1912.[1] In Volumes 3 and 4, Lavinia Dock detailed her personal knowledge of the emergence of nursing in the northern hemisphere, Europe, parts of Asia, Australia, and New Zealand, and published many photographs of the nurses she believed important in that process. ICN founder Ethel Gordon Fenwick, and her associate, Margaret Breay, wrote the first official history of the ICN in 1923.[2] In 1967, ICN Secretary Daisy Bridges, published her very useful history of the first 65 years of the International Council of Nurses.[3] About 20 years later, in 1989, ICN Secretary Sheila Quinn updated the Bridges history by concentrating on the era of rapid ICN expansion during the 1970s and 1980s.[4] In between, ICN writers published historical accounts in International Nursing Review and occasional pieces in national nursing journals.

All these useful histories were written by ICN "insiders," which means that their perspective on the ICN was positive and organizational conflict or failure could well be understated or unexamined. We understand that these works tell us what the ICN most wanted told about itself at the time they were written. Equally important, they might omit matters insiders thought either unimportant or inappropriate to record as history. An important function of these histories was to help the ICN create its chosen identity. And, indeed, it is through these histories that most of us 'know what we think we know' about the ICN's past. For us as researchers, the histories constituted valuable sources against which we could compare primary materials from the ICN archives and other sources. They help establish or check the general chronology. The histories also generated an archive of their own; the correspondence between ICN leaders and the authors of the histories often illuminated debates otherwise hard to understand. And, of course, all the histories include photographs that are a treasure in themselves.

One could now ask whether still another history of the ICN is needed. Naturally, we think so. The present-day ICN's openness to historical research by "outsiders" assures a different history from people influenced by a different set of experiences and goals. Nursing did not move from darkness to light with the aid of Nightingale's lamp and the ICN did not trace a straight path from the vision of Ethel Gordon Fenwick, Lavinia Dock, and Germany's Agnes Karll to become an international voice for world nursing. The devil and the delight is in the details of the story—in the ambiguities, the conflicts, and even in the missing evidence. A nuanced, contextual history informed by current scholarship will find its own useful place in the scheme of things.

Finally, we faced some basic issues in doing this history. Perhaps the most problematic is who we, the authors, are. Three of us are from the United States, one from Canada, one from Great Britain, and one from the Netherlands. All white women, and, we acknowledge, a rather Anglo-Eurocentric group. On the other hand, we are also all well-trained and experienced historians representing wide interests in relevant historical scholarship. We are sensitive to the fact that we, in our persons, reflect the Anglo-European origins of the ICN. But we take responsibility for our interpretation, with its strengths and weaknesses, and combining that with the importance of doing the project, justify our credibility to do justice to the work. Of course, we do not delude ourselves by thinking that an all-encompassing, eclectically embracing account of any organization as complex and variegated as the ICN is really possible. We certainly do not claim that ours can be that. What we do hope is that this account will stimulate awareness of the rich historical possibilities in the history of nursing in the 20th century and will prompt others to research and write their own interpretations. In the end, the story of the ICN holds a mirror to the 20th century; its members and leaders, with their hopes and struggles, teach us and broaden our understanding of who we are.

## ENDNOTES

1. M. Adelaide Nutting and Lavinia L. Dock: *A History of Nursing* In Two Volumes (New York and London: G.P. Putnam's Sons, 1907) and Lavinia L. Dock, *A History of Nursing* Volumes III and IV (New York and London: G.P. Putnam's Sons, 1912).

2. Margaret Breay and Ethel Gordon Fenwick: "History of the International Council of Nurses, 1899–1925," compiled from official documents. Written about 1929, this was privately published. Archives, International Council of Nurses, Geneva, Switzerland.
3. Daisy Caroline Bridges: *A History of the International Council of Nurses 1899–1964* (Philadelphia and Toronto: J.B. Lippincott Company, 1967).
4. Dame Sheila Quinn: *ICN Past and Present* (Middlesex, England: Scutari Press, 1989).

# *Above All Other Things—Unity*

### NANCY J. TOMES
### *with Geertje Boschma*

In 1899, a British suffragist and nurse named Ethel Gordon Fenwick had the bold idea that nurses of various countries should unite in an international nursing organization. She believed that by linking their infant national societies, each struggling to improve its professional status, nurses would strengthen their vocational cause at home as well as promote the highest standards abroad. In elevating the profession of nursing, so closely identified with the female gender, the ardent feminist Fenwick thought that an international coalition of nurses would also elevate the position of women around the world.

Fenwick presented this idea to her fellow British nurses at the 1899 annual meeting of the Matrons' Council of Great Britain and Ireland. Many of its members had just come from a meeting of the International Council of Women (ICW), a coalition of women's suffrage, reform, and professional associations from Europe and the United States. Inspired by a day-long meeting of the ICW's Nursing Section, at which nurses from around the world had presented papers, Fenwick proposed that the Matrons' Council undertake the task of forming an International Council of Nurses (ICN). She exhorted the assembled nurse leaders, "The nursing profession above all things requires organization; nurses, above all other things, require to be united."

If nurses were to do their best for the sick, Fenwick continued, they had to have a uniform and exacting system of training. "The experience of the past," she observed, "has proved that these results can never be obtained by any profession unless it is united in its demands for the necessary reform, and by union alone can the necessary strength be obtained." Fenwick did not find daunting the task of uniting nurses from different countries in a common course of action, for in her words,

[T]he work of nursing is one of humanity all the world over, and it is one therefore which appeals to women of every land without distinction of

1

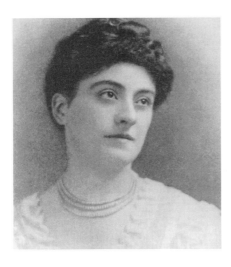

**FIGURE 1-1**
*Ethel Gordon Fenwick, founder of the International Council of Nurses. From LL Dock, History of Nursing, Vol 3, 1912.*

class or degree or nationality. The work in which nurses are engaged in other countries is precisely the same as that in our own.

Thus, she concluded, the "need for nursing progress" and the "principals of organization" were identical the world over.[1] The Matrons' Council approved Fenwick's plan for the ICN and appointed a Provisional Committee to do the necessary formation work. Over the next year, the committee drafted a constitution for the organization and circulated it among nursing leaders and organizations in Europe and North America. The constitution was approved at the next meeting of the Provisional Committee in July 1900. Under its terms, the ICN elected its first slate of officers: an English president, Ethel Gordon Fen-

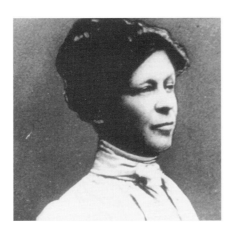

**FIGURE 1-2**
*Lavinia L. Dock, Honorary Secretary of the International Council of Nurses, 1900 to 1923. From Lynaugh Collection, Bryn Mawr, PA.*

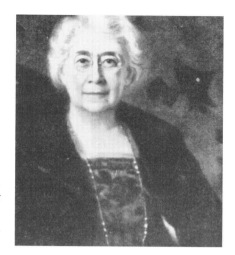

**FIGURE 1-3**
*Mary Agnes Snively, Honorary Treasurer, International Council of Nurses, 1900 to 1904. From Bridges, History of the International Council of Nurses, 1967.*

wick; an American secretary, Lavinia Dock; and a Canadian treasurer, Agnes Snively. Plans were made to hold the first formal meeting of the ICN in Buffalo, New York, in September 1901.

As this oft-told account of its founding makes evident, the ICN, in its original incarnation, was essentially an Anglo-American enterprise. Although individuals from Germany and Denmark actively participated in its early affairs, nurses from England and her colonies, past and present, dominated the ICN's ideals and organization during its first decade. Thus, the early history of the ICN was tied up with the development of what was then called the "women's movement" in England and the United States. This chapter looks first at the Anglo-American scene, which gave rise to the ICN idea, and the initial goals of its leadership, which was dominated by nurses from England and her colonies, past and present. Against this backdrop, it then considers the very different development of nursing in Germany, as a case study of the ICN's early concerns, with particular emphasis on the career of Agnes Karll.

## The 19th-Century Women's Movement

The ICN grew out of the upwelling of female-directed reforms in 19th-century England and the United States. Beginning in the late 1700s, women from the middle and upper classes became involved in a wide spectrum of charitable and improving activities. This women's movement encompassed vibrant crusades for women's education, suffrage, poverty relief, foreign missions, temperance, and prison reform. Their crusades were premised on the idea that all women shared a fundamental identity derived from their unique biological and social destiny. As historian Nancy Cott wrote, "Nineteenth-century women's consistent usage of the singular *woman* symbolized, in a word, the unity of the female sex." They believed in the proposition, as Cott put it, "that all women have one cause, one movement."[2] This new sense of gender consciousness and desire to partici-pate *as women* in public life grew out of a vast array of economic and social changes.[3] In both England and the United States, the rise of commercial capitalism transformed the roles of women; as shops and factories replaced home manufacturing, and more families moved from farm to city, a new domestic ideal emerged among the affluent. The productive labors of the 18th-century housewife gave way to a new bourgeois cult of domesticity that defined women's identity in terms of their moral and emotional duties within the family. Nineteenth-century gender stereotypes highlighted the opposition of certain male and female traits. Men were considered rational, aggressive, and easily overpowered by their base natures, whereas women were seen as emotional, nurturant, and having a keener moral sensibility.

Ironically, the increasing emphasis on women's domestic duties cre-ated the basis for a greater sense of their common social and political interests outside the home. To begin with, the new domesticity required that women receive more education, because ignorant women could not exercise the proper influence over their children or husbands. As the educational opportunities for boys expanded to meet the need for a more highly skilled work force, girls were able to profit as well, particularly in the United States, where public education came to be seen as a democratic right. With each generation, more women possessed the basic skills of reading and writing essential to forming and voicing political opinions.

Second, the growing uniformity of women's domestic roles created a new sense of unity among them. Despite growing extremes of wealth, the conventions of the cult of domesticity flattened the sense of difference among women in the middle and upper classes. Most affluent women mar-ried and set up households that followed a similar routine; they supervised shopping and servants, they bore and reared children, they attended church and paid calls. Despite growing class differences, many women's daily rou-tines had a sameness that reflected their new roles in industrial society.

Religion was another force instilling a common sense of purpose among the predominantly Protestant women of the upper classes. Amidst fierce competitions between its evangelical and nonevangelical camps, Anglo-American Protestantism flourished in the 1800s. Denominations expanded their buildings, their memberships, their educational institu-tions, and their outreach programs to create what historians have termed the *benevolent empire*. The language of Protestantism suffused science, do-mestic politics, and international affairs. At the same time, church life became a much more exclusively female domain; women outnumbered men as converts and as church members. A shared sense of Christian purpose became a powerful force unifying women from different regional and social backgrounds.

The resurgent Protestantism of the 19th century prompted an extraordinary outpouring of reformist zeal. From the pulpit and the pages of religious periodicals, Protestants heard that true Christians, female as well as male, had an obligation to do God's work on earth, to eliminate sin, and spread the gospel. Beginning in the early 1800s, women joined both same-sex and gender-integrated reform societies dedicated to bringing Christianity to the poor and to "heathens," fostering abstinence from alcohol, and putting an end to slavery both at home and abroad. In the process, they learned how to raise money, run meetings, give speeches, and petition legislators for their various causes.

To promote a sense of common interest among women from different backgrounds, women reformers relied on what they assumed were shared experiences of childbirth and child nurture, devotion to home and family, and Christian duty. Ostensibly free from the commercial strivings and biological urges that troubled their menfolk, they felt able to act as the conscience of the community. Catharine Beecher, one of the premier voices of the women's movement, wrote, in a passage that could just as easily have applied to English women,

> To American women, more than to any others on earth, is committed the exalted privilege of extending over the world those blessed influences, which are to renovate degraded man, and "to clothe all climes with beauty."[4]

In retrospect, the convictions that these women reformers held about the unity and influence of womanhood are difficult to understand. The supposedly universal female character that they invoked was, in fact, the product of a distinctively white, middle-class, Protestant culture. At the very time that this sense of gender unity developed, women's lives were becoming more and more differentiated by class and race. The existence of the middle-class lady was made possible only by the labors of the working-class servant, the immigrant, the factory girl, and the African American slave, for whom the cult of domesticity had little relevance.[5]

Yet, however flawed it appears in retrospect, the 19th-century conception of womanhood still fostered powerful new forms of identification among different groups of women. The conviction that all members of their gender shared essential traits and experiences helped affluent women to identify with their poor, enslaved, and foreign-born counterparts. Their reform agendas reflected the maternalistic assumption that educated and refined women had a special obligation to uplift their less privileged sisters. As we shall see, this ambivalent mixture of identification and maternalism, or what one historian has called the "relations of rescue," carried over into the crusade for international nursing uplift.[6]

## Missionaries and Suffragists

The ICN fused together two distinct strands of the larger 19th-century women's movement: the missionary movement and the women's suffrage crusade. From the former, the early ICN leadership inherited a long tradition of cross-cultural relationships among women of different races and religion, which allowed them to define their own identity in comparison to a less progressive "other." From the suffrage movement, the ICN nurses adopted the belief that women-led organizations were the only route to true female autonomy and professional improvement.

The ICN built upon almost a century of Anglo-American missionary activity. Among the earliest good works women embarked on was carrying the gospel of Christianity to "heathen" women in foreign lands. Women formed mite or cent societies to pay the costs of sending missionaries overseas. Religious newspapers and magazines, which middle-class women read more extensively than their secular counterparts, chronicled the adventures of foreign missionaries in great detail. In the first half of the century, women missionaries were the wives of ministers and doctors sent overseas to found churches and clinics; their efforts to spread the "gospel of gentility," as historian Jane Hunter has termed it, fascinated their counterparts back home.[7] For example, the three wives of Adoniram Judson, the first missionary to Thailand, became celebrated heroines among American Baptist women. In the late 1800s, single women trained as physicians and schoolteachers joined the missionary ranks. By the 1890s, women comprised 60% of all mission workers in the United States.[8]

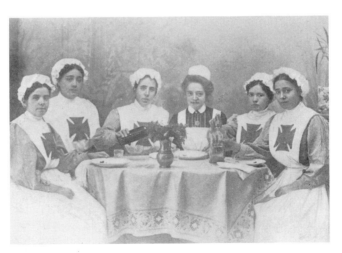

*FIGURE 1-4*
*A group of Spanish probationer nurses at the turn of the 20th century. From LL Dock, History of Nursing, Vol. 4, 1912.*

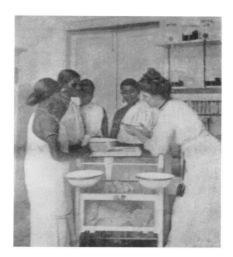

**FIGURE 1-5**
*Instruction in nursing in India—about 1895. From LL Dock, History of Nursing, Vol. 4, 1912.*

For Anglo-American women, the missionary impulse expressed and reinforced a strong sense of moral and social superiority.[9] Contemplating the life of native women, and the varied travails of foot binding, child marriage, polygamy, and suttee they faced, gave Christian women a pleasurable sense of their own exalted place in society. Besides the vicarious thrill of reading about the hedonistic sins of the unconverted, this involvement with mission work brought Anglo-American women to think of an imagined community of women around the world. As we shall see, the ICN built a similar sense of imagined community around the shared identity of woman as nurse.[10]

The second strand of the women's movement that even more directly gave rise to the ICN was the women's suffrage movement, which began in the United States in the 1840s, and slightly later in Great Britain. It was a natural extension of one of the great political developments of the 19th century: the extension of suffrage to all men, regardless of their class or education level. In the United States, universal white men's suffrage was accomplished in the early 1800s; at the close of the Civil War, the vote was extended to black men as well (although the right was soon abridged by state laws). In Great Britain, a series of reform bills expanded men's suffrage dramatically between 1832 and 1884, although it did not become universal until 1918, the same year women over the age of 30 gained the vote. As the right to vote was extended to more and more men, its denial to women of equivalent class or educational status became all the more galling to a growing number of women.

The immediate precipitant for the women's suffrage movement was the experience of women abolitionists in the United States. Beginning in the 1820s, many middle-class Northern women were drawn into the antislavery movement for reasons quite similar to their attraction to foreign missionary work. To their way of thinking, the plight of the enslaved Africans represented a threat to the nation's moral fabric. As white Christian women, they felt a particular call to rescue slave women from their masters' disregard of their moral virtue and their sacred duties as wives and mothers.

But as the women antislavery activists soon realized, limitations on their own political and economic rights hobbled what they could do for those they deemed less fortunate. The prevailing assumptions about a distinctive female moral authority did not ensure them an equal voice even among their fellow reformers. The bitter experience of being barred from the 1840 World's Antislavery Convention in London led directly to the first Women's Rights Convention in 1848, when a group of disgruntled women reformers met at Seneca Falls, New York, to discuss grievances. Drafting a Declaration of Principles patterned on the American Declaration of Independence, they argued that, in terms of legal and political rights, women were no better than the slaves they sought to aid through the antislavery movement. Among their many demands, the Seneca Falls participants put forward the then radical proposition that women be given the ballot.[11]

In England, the women's suffrage movement developed around the same time period. The Chartist movement included the vote for women on its reform agenda in the 1840s. In 1867, John Stuart Mill submitted the first bill for women's suffrage to Parliament. Its defeat led to the formation of local suffrage societies in England and Scotland. A National Society for Women's Suffrage was founded in 1869.[12]

But, as of the late 1800s, the women's suffrage movement in both the United States and England still found only limited support even among reformers. The vast majority of middle- and upper-class women, including those active in charitable and reform work, continued to believe that women did not need the vote in order to bring their distinctively female virtues to bear on the public sphere. Not until a new generation of leaders, with a professional and international agenda in mind, came to the fore at the end of the century did the cause of suffrage, and the closely allied cause of professional nursing, begin to gain more ground.

## The Origins of Women's Internationalism

In the latter decades of the 19th century, the Anglo-American women's movement became increasingly international in scope. A long tradition of colonial enterprises and foreign mission work acquainted British and American women with the lives of women in such exotic places as China, India, and Burma. Likewise, the Anglo-American antislavery movement fostered an international level of interest and collaboration. For a variety of technological and economic reasons, Anglo-American women became even more aware of their ties to one another, and to women in other countries, during the last quarter of the 19th century.

This sense of interconnectedness was helped by dramatic improvements in both transportation and communication. Within nations and continents, the expansion of railroads facilitated the exchange of people and goods. The opening of the Suez Canal in 1869 dramatically reduced the time needed to voyage from Europe to Southeast Asia. With the introduction of steam-powered ocean liners in the 1880s, the cost in time and money of travel around the world declined. For example, a voyage from the United States to Europe that once might have taken several months could be accomplished in a matter of weeks.

The laying of international telegraph cables in the 1860s, and the development of wireless telegraphy in the late 1890s, allowed ever more rapid transmission of economic and political news. Commercial telephone service became available in large American and European cities in the late 1870s. The development of cheaper forms of papermaking and printing increased the number of newspapers, magazines, and books available to disseminate news about other nations and cultures. In all these ways, the world seemed to be coming closer together in the late 1800s.

The extension of European colonialism also created new links among different parts of the world. Innovations in transport and communication, coupled with the wealth generated by industrialization, fostered an aggressive European presence, both militarily and economically, in Africa, India, Latin America, and Asia. The British dominated the late 19th century imperial order, but after 1870, a newly united Germany became an increasingly powerful competitor. France, Italy, and after 1898, the United States, also built significant overseas empires in the waning years of the 19th century.

The wealth of raw materials provided by colonial possessions, combined with technological innovations in steel and chemical manufacturing, food processing, and energy production, fueled the maturation of industrial capitalism in both Europe and the United States. The volume of international trade increased dramatically in the late 1800s. Small family businesses gave way to large corporations that sought to control national and international markets to their advantage. Professional skills in banking, law, and engineering became increasingly vital to large-scale economic activities. In economic and organizational terms, this was a period of growing consolidation and bureaucratization.

The same spirit of interconnectedness animated the social and cultural life of the period. Starting with the celebrated Crystal Palace exhibition in 1851, world's fairs and international congresses became increasingly popular. Exhibitions held in various Western European and American cities allowed inventors and manufacturers the opportunity to show off their latest wares, whereas civic and cultural groups called attention to the growth of art, culture, and benevolence.

Professional groups staged international meetings to exchange information and build solidarity. Physicians began holding periodic International Medical Congresses in 1867; other groups, from public health officials and ophthalmologists to homeopathic physicians and statisticians, soon followed suit. Although dedicated to the pursuit of supposedly universal scientific truths, such gatherings also promoted a strong sense of rivalry among the intellectual and professional elites of the different nations.

Simultaneously, the foreign missionary movement expanded rapidly during these same years. As Western nations extended their economic and political control of their overseas colonies, foreign missionaries supplied the personnel and the funds to extend Western cultural influences as well. With funds solicited from their loyal constituencies at home, many Protestant denominations built churches, schools, and hospitals in an effort to Christianize and civilize the native inhabitants. The number of women involved in both the domestic and overseas operations of the missions work increased dramatically; as one male missionary officer referred to it, the foreign missions represented "a great uprising of Christian women in behalf of their sex."[13]

## The International Council of Women

Women's organizations showed the same strong impulse to internationalize during these decades. By the late 1870s and 1880s, vibrant national organizations dedicated to women's causes such as temperance and suffrage existed in a number of countries; the next logical step was to forge alliances across national lines. The World Woman's Christian Temperance Union (WCTU), formed in 1884, provided the first example of the new women's internationalism.[14] At the suggestion of Frances Willard, President of the American WCTU, a Boston woman, Mary Clement Leavitt, began to travel the globe to forge an international coalition of temperance organizations.[15]

The same year that Willard conceived of the World's WCTU, the American suffragist Elizabeth Cady Stanton had the idea of founding an international coalition of women's suffrage advocates. On a trip to Europe in 1882 to 1883, Stanton broached the idea at a meeting of leaders from various national suffrage groups in Liverpool, England. They formed a Committee on Correspondence—invoking, as at Seneca Falls, the language of the American Revolution with its like-named committees—to develop the idea. They decided to hold the first meeting of the new international group in 1888, to commemorate the 40th anniversary of the Seneca Falls Convention and the founding of the first American suffrage organization.[16]

But as the meeting drew nearer, the conception of the group to be formed changed significantly. Instead of an international suffrage organization, it was to include, in the words of the American feminist May Wright Sewall, "women workers along all lines of social, intellectual, moral or civic progress and reform." Supposedly, Susan B. Anthony, Stanton's long-time collaborator in the suffrage cause, suggested the broader conception of the group as one more befitting the wide-ranging scope of contemporary women's activities. In addition, deemphasizing the vexed question of political rights would allow women's groups that shied away from the suffrage issue to show a sense of solidarity with other women reformers.[17] The ICW met from March 25 to April 1, 1888, at Albaugh's Opera House in Washington, DC. Appointed chair of the meeting, Susan B. Anthony presided over 49 delegates representing 53 different organizations from 10 nations, Canada, France, England, Scotland, Ireland, India, Norway, Denmark, Finland, and the United States. In the opening address, the venerable Elizabeth Cady Stanton explained why it was that women from such different parts of the world would find it easy to communicate with one another.

"We do not feel that you are strangers and foreigners," Stanton told the assembled delegates, "for the women of all nationalities, in the artificial distinctions of sex, have a universal sense of injustice, that forms a common bond of union between them." Eloquently invoking the many forms of injustice against their sex, she claimed, "Whether our feet are compressed in iron shoes, our faces hidden with veils and masks, whether yoked with cows to draw the plow through its furrows, or classed with idiots, lunatics, and criminals in the laws and constitutions of the state, the principle is the same, for the humiliations of spirit are as real as the visible badges of servitude." Nations might differ in "government, religion, laws, and social customs," she noted, but for woman, the "subordination in all nations is the rule of her being." She concluded that different languages and creeds need not divide the women of the world, because "through suffering we have learned the open sesame to the hearts of each other."[18]

In the days that followed, the delegates heard a variety of papers on issues of special interest to women, including temperance, suffrage, and social purity. By the close of the meeting, the delegates had approved two constitutions, one for the National Council of Women (NCW) for the United States, the second for the International Council. The preamble of the Constitution of the ICW explained the goals of the new association: that "the women of all nations" had banded together "to promote the highest good of the family and of the state" in a federation of women "of all races, nations, creeds and classes." Despite the reference to many creeds, the ultimate aim of the ICW was cast in unmistakably Christian terms: to apply "the Golden Rule to society, custom and law: 'Do unto others as ye would that they should do unto you.'"[19] The foreign delegates returned to their countries and began forming their own national councils, modeled on the American one. The idea was to create a chain of women stretching upward from local organizations through state and regional associations, which would federate with the NCW. Each national council would then be federated with the international council. By the first quinquennial conference of the ICW, held in 1893 at the Columbian Exposition in Chicago, six nations had national councils in the planning stages.

Meeting concurrently with the ICW, the NCW of the United States organized a World Congress of Representative Women for the 1893 Chicago exposition. A circular sent to women's groups in "every country of the civilized world," in the words of its organizers, brought out thousands of participants at the meetings of the World Congress. More than 600 women participated in the discussion of topics such as women's suffrage, temperance, and conditions of labor.[20]

## Beginnings of the International Nursing Idea

Among the thousands of women involved in the Chicago congress was Ethel Gordon Fenwick. Fenwick, having been instrumental in the founding of the British Nurses Association (BNA) in 1887, was chosen to represent her nation's nurses as president of the British Nursing Section. Visiting the United States in 1892 to help plan the meeting, she thought it a good idea to try to make the acquaintance of American nursing leaders. Fenwick recalled in 1907, "Matrons of hospitals were in those days not well known to each other." So she "asked a lady in Chicago a question she would have no need to ask now, namely, who were the great leaders of nursing in the American continent." The American woman told Fenwick to contact Isabel Hampton, the head of the Johns Hopkins School of Nursing, and Fenwick immediately wrote her, suggesting a meeting. In response, Hampton invited Fenwick to stop in Baltimore on her way home from Chicago. Fenwick spent several days at Hopkins, discussing the state of nursing with both Hampton and her assistant superintendent, Lavinia L. Dock. In retrospect, Fenwick felt that "the seed of the International Nursing movement, now so full of vitality, was then sown."[21]

At the time of this 1892 meeting, nursing leaders in England and the United States shared a common historical background and faced similar challenges. The nursing professions in both countries stemmed from the hospital reform movement started by Florence Nightingale on her return from the Crimean War in the late 1850s. This daughter of the English gentry had successfully demonstrated that women nurses drawn from the "better ranks" of society could elevate the moral and medical standards of English hospitals. Although she thought of nursing as a religious vocation rather than a secular profession, Nightingale helped transform it into a respectable career for the daughters of middle-class Britons and Americans.

The founding of hospital training schools based on Nightingale's principles accelerated rapidly in the decades after 1860. The new schools fulfilled two critical functions in the 1870s and 1880s: in exchange for training as nurses, young women provided hospitals with an expanded corps of skilled workers. Both the nurses and the hospital managers benefited from the arrangement. But by the 1890s, the rapid expansion of hospital training schools had created some serious dilemmas of growth on both sides of the Atlantic.

First, the educational aims of the hospital schools were subordinated to the hospital's need for labor. The long hours that student nurses were expected to put in on the wards left little time for concentrated study. Efforts to improve the educational content of their training often met resistance from hospital superintendents and trustees primarily concerned with keeping labor costs low. Second, the program of training varied enormously from school to school. Although some schools set high standards for admission and graduation, others required relatively little but labor from their pupils. By the 1890s, the nursing market was being flooded by nurses with hospital diplomas representing enormous variations in training. Last but not least, nurses who completed hospital training enjoyed no professional or legal preference over the many women who continued to acquire their nursing experience outside the hospital.

By the 1890s, nursing leaders in both England and the United States began to organize as a way to solve these various problems. In England, Fenwick founded the BNA in 1887 to promote the interests of hospital-trained nurses over their untrained competitors. The Matrons' Council, founded in 1894, provided the heads of the hospital schools a forum in which to discuss shared problems and formulate common educational standards. In the United States, alumnae associations of the various training schools affiliated in 1896; they became officially known as the American Nurses Association (ANA) in 1911. The American Society of Superintendents of Training Schools for Nurses (ASSTSN), which became the National League of Nursing Education (NLNE), was founded in 1893.

From these early organizational efforts, a common set of solutions to professional nursing problems began to emerge. Higher educational standards would be set for incoming nursing students. Before probationers went on the ward, they needed a preliminary course of instruction. The curriculum must be made uniform and, to accommodate the preliminary course, should ideally be extended from 2 to 3 years. Once the title "trained nurse" became more uniform, it needed to be accorded more exclusivity; only nurses who had completed a rigorous course of training and passed a final examination should be allowed to use it. The final step would be registration. The state would certify or register hospital-trained nurses the same way it licensed physicians, and make it illegal for untrained competitors to invoke the title of trained or registered nurse.

Late 19th-century nursing leaders attached extraordinary importance to this final step of registration. For them, registration held out the same promise that the vote did for women in general. As they well knew, physicians effectively used the power of the state to secure their own professional status through licensing laws that forced out untrained or unorthodox practitioners. Following the same model, nursing leaders hoped to make registration a tool for elevating the status of their own profession. If, in order to qualify for the title "trained nurse," student nurses had to take specific courses and pass more demanding examinations, hospital training schools would have to adjust their admission standards and curriculum accordingly.[22]

In the 1890s, the agenda of professional uplift was already being discussed by British and American nursing leaders, but the means to realize their goals were still unclear. Although the campaign to raise educational standards and secure professional recognition absorbed the heads of the elite training schools, it held far less appeal for the vast number of nurses simply trying to secure a living, or the hospital superintendents, trustees, and physicians anxious to secure a cheap and docile labor force. The Anglo-American nursing elite saw itself as a beleaguered minority calling for higher standards in the midst of a commercialized wilderness.

Fenwick saw the virtues of international combination largely in terms of strengthening the reformers' positions within their respective nations. By sharing ideas and strategies, they might better craft their national crusades to uplift nursing. If one country achieved a superior educational standard or legal protection for nurses, all the rest might cite it in their own battles, appealing to the spirit of national rivalry. In this fashion, international communication and cooperation would advance the whole of the nursing profession.

Fenwick put this strategy to work immediately after her very first visit to the United States. In an article published in the *Nursing Record,* she recounted some of "the lessons which I think we may learn from our American sisters on Nursing matters." Chief among these lessons was her conclusion that in the United States, "Nursing is looked upon as a profession, while in the United Kingdom it is really treated as a trade." She chided her English colleagues with the observation that "we shall find amongst American Nurses, as a class, a much better and higher professional feeling than prevails in this country."[23]

The second quinquennial meeting of the ICW, held in London in July 1899, gave Fenwick the ideal opportunity to pursue the international strategy further. She was appointed convener of the ICW's Professional Section, which organized 16 sessions on women's participation in various professions. One of the sessions was a day-long meeting on nursing that touched on all the issues on the nurse reformers' agenda, from preliminary training of new pupils to state registration of graduate nurses. The tenor of those discussions well illustrates the outlook of the early nurse leaders who soon came together to form the ICN.

The first two papers concerned nursing in two British colonies, New Zealand and South Africa. Grace Neill of the Wellington Hospital gave an overview of the "Professional Training and Status of Nurses," which stressed the value of preliminary education, admission examinations, and certification of nurses. Neill noted that possessing the vote was of immeasurable value to New Zealand nurses. "You can have no idea what a difference it will make to your interest and your status when once it is an accepted fact that women and men have equal electoral rights as citizens and subjects of the Queen," she concluded.[24]

Next, M. H. Watkins reported on the operation of the 1892 Nurse Registration Act passed in South Africa, the first of its kind. To be registered, nurses had to pass an examination administered twice a year by two physicians. Not surprisingly, Watkins portrayed the law as a great success; she reported that

> Registration has had a markedly good effect in the Colony—1st, by raising the standard of education for nurses; 2nd, in raising the status of nurses; 3rd, in awakening ambition in nurses; and 4th, in affording, by their published Register, an opportunity to the public of knowing that the nurse they engage is duly qualified, an opportunity of which, I am glad to say, many avail themselves.[25]

From the United States, the participants in the Nursing Section heard a glowing report on the value of associated alumnae societies. A paper written by Isabel Hampton Robb, then head of the National Associated Alumnae of the United States, outlined the importance of these societies as building blocks of nursing organization. She described how in the United States, the "commercial spirit" led to the proliferation of low-quality nursing schools, endangering the credentials of women who had "devoted years to learning their profession." In response, the better schools formed alumnae associations to promote their interests. Robb explained,

> The present age is one of organization, and graduate nurses are finding that, as a class, they are not exempt from difficulties and problems against which individual efforts are of no avail, and learning by experience that progress, improvement, and ideals, can be attained only by combined efforts with unity of purpose and centralization of means, have organized themselves into Alumnae Associations.[26]

In the discussions following these various papers, participants compared notes on the state of nursing education, state registration, and the general status of the profession in their respective countries. Throughout their remarks, there was a sense of agreement that nurses must band together to improve their situation. At the same time, many expressed concern that professional standards not become mechanical. The best nurses, they agreed, had a quality of character or "refinement" that could not be measured by examinations. New Zealander Neill urged, "Teach nurses the beauty of a quiet, reposeful nature; such a nature is in itself balm to the convalescing."[27]

Even Lavinia Dock, one of the most tireless American advocates of higher standards for nursing, wondered, "Has there been, perhaps, a tendency in the nurses' teaching to leave the individuality of the patient as a suffering human atom too far out of sight?" She added, "It has occurred to me that when we are sometimes chagrined by the preference of patient or physician for what we call an 'old-fashioned nurse,' it simply means that in a crude, blundering way they are seeking the 'ever womanly' which in the alert, up-to-date, soldier-like nurse, in full armor, though surely present, is sometimes hidden out of sight."[28]

But no one at the Nursing Section meeting expressed any reservations about the concept that nursing progress rested on further organization. Individualism and self-interest were condemned as behind the times; nursing unity and organization would only promote the best care of the sick and the higher ideals of humanity. Mary Agnes Snively of the Toronto General Hospital summed up the advantages of forming societies: "The greater strength which comes from union; the mutual help, protection, and inspiration, which intercourse imparts: the increased facilities and incentives which organization gives for holding fast that which has been already attained, and of elevating or improving the standard of work, thereby adding to the dignity of the profession."[29]

## The Birth of the ICN

At the close of the ICW meeting, the Matrons' Council of Great Britain and Ireland held a banquet in honor of May Wright Sewall, the American ICW leader. "Realizing the importance of the occasion, and the benefit to all nurses, of personal intercourse, and exchange of experiences between nurses of various nations," the Council invited the American and Canadian nurses who had attended the congress as well.[30] At that banquet, the idea of an international association of nurses was first discussed in an informal fashion.[31] The next day, some 200 women reconvened at Number 20, Hanover Square for the Second Annual Conference of the Matron's Council of Great Britain and Ireland. Chair Isla Stewart presided over the large group, which included the foreign nurses who came for the ICW Congress.

Coming straight from the exhilarating women's congress, Ethel Gordon Fenwick had little difficulty convincing those assembled that forming an International Council of Nurses was an admirable idea. "If the poet's dream of the brotherhood of man is ever to be fulfilled, surely a sisterhood

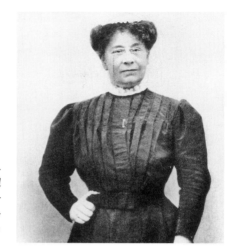

**FIGURE 1-6**
*Isla Stewart, President of the Matron's Council of Great Britain and Ireland and Matron of St. Bartholomew's Hospital, London. From LL Dock, History of Nursing, Vol. 3, 1912.*

of nurses is an international idea, and one in which the women of all nations, therefore, could be asked and expected to join," she proclaimed.[32] As the minutes of the ICN recorded, "The idea was cordially received by all and the nurses who had taken part in the Congress formed themselves into a provisional committee to arrange the details of organization."[33]

The Matrons' Council was then addressed by May Wright Sewall. Although not herself a nurse, Sewall's remarks to the group summed up the unique characteristics of the nursing sisterhood her colleague Fenwick envisioned. Sewall began by stating her conviction that a nurse's work "lifted her out of the limitations that beset other occupations" because it essentially denied the importance of nationality. Nurses did not, she observed, "enquire to what nationality the man or woman belongs whom you are called to nurse" nor did a fever ask that question "before taking possession of its victim." Diseases might vary in different climates, yet they made no distinction between a "Duchess" or a "drudge." Sewall expressed her belief that nurses, more than other women professionals, had the power to "lift themselves out of the clutches of prejudice into the freer realm where the International Idea was born and must expand."[34] Sewall's speech outlined several themes that would reappear frequently in the ICN's work to come: the idea that the universal characteristics of the body in health and disease formed a natural unity in the nurse's work; that nursing was apart from or above politics; that the ethos of nursing should be a counterpoint to the spirit of nationalism with its potential for discord and violence; and that "female" virtues of cooperation and service, as exemplified by nursing, could balance and even transcend the "male" vices of competition and aggression.

Inspired by Fenwick and Sewall, the Provisional Committee moved quickly to organize the new ICN. The British contingent on the committee met that summer to draft the constitution, which they then forwarded for comments to the nursing associations already extant in the United States, Holland, and Denmark. In July 1900, an enlarged Provisional Committee met to consider the suggestions and criticisms they had received, and the first constitution was approved, which, with relatively few amendments, served the ICN until 1925.[35]

The new ICN drew heavily on the ICW plan of organization. The preamble of its 1900 constitution paraphrased the 1888 constitution of the ICW. It read, "We nurses of all nations, sincerely believing that the best good of our Profession will be advanced by greater unity of thought, sympathy and purpose, do hereby band ourselves in a confederation of workers to further the efficient care of the sick, and to secure the honour and the interests of the Nursing Profession."[36]

Like the ICW, the ICN was organized around National Councils of Nurses, representing the different nursing organizations of each country. Starting with local alumnae associations, the lines of organization proceeded upward to the national nursing associations, which were joined in a national nursing council. The national council would then federate with the international body, paying yearly dues equivalent to 1£ sterling per delegate for its support. The president of each national council became a vice president in the ICN. In addition, each national council had the right to send four representatives to the ICN Grand Council. An executive committee, formed of past and present officers, dealt with more immediate tasks of governing the association. Meetings of the whole ICN were to be held at 5-year intervals; only those nurses affiliated with societies belonging to the ICN could vote at its public congresses.

In commenting on the proposed constitution, Lavinia Dock suggested appointing two German women to represent that nation on the council. The Provisional Committee decided instead "to follow the procedure of the International Council of Women" and reserve the position of honorary vice president for such countries as had not yet formed a national council. The ICN Executive Committee could select an honorary vice president to represent them.

Another question that prompted debate during the drafting of the constitution concerned whether past officers of the ICN should continue to have a vote on the Executive Committee. Lavinia Dock thought this practice was "contrary to democratic principles and likely to make trouble," and, according to the minutes, "considerable discussion ensued." Ultimately, the group decided that the ICN could not afford to be so democratic. The other members of the committee felt that Great Britain and other European countries were behind the United States and Canada in nursing organization and that, unless the constitution allowed for some continuity of leadership and policy in its early years, the council would every 5 years become completely disorganized. Once again, the ICW provided a precedent; the fact that it "had found it desirable to retain the service of its past presidents" was offered in support of the ICN doing the same. The Provisional Committee decided that experience was essential to keeping the fledgling organization together. Not only were former officers allowed to keep their votes, but all members of the Provisional Committee were designated as Foundation Members and given the same privilege.[37]

At the conclusion of the 1900 meeting of the Provisional Committee, the constitution was adopted and the first officers of the association, President Ethel Gordon Fenwick, Secretary Lavinia L. Dock, and Treasurer Mary Agnes Snively, were elected. Rather than wait 5 years for their next meeting, the officers agreed to accept the offer, made by the Nurses Association of Buffalo, New York, to host a meeting of the ICN in September 1901, in conjunction with the Pan-American Exposition. Fenwick and her compatriots believed there was no time to be wasted in building support for the organization, so Dock and Snively immediately set to work making arrangements for the 1901 Buffalo Congress.

## The Buffalo Congress, 1901

The first Congress of the ICN convened on September 14, 1901, in the hall of the Women's Educational and Industrial Union building in Niagara Square. Its meeting was held in conjunction with the Nurses' Associated Alumnae of the United States, the ASSTSN, and the Spanish-American Order of War Nurses. As part of the Pan-American Exposition, the American nursing societies organized the Third International Congress of Nurses (the first two having been held in Chicago in 1893 and London in 1899), to follow the ICN Congress.

In her opening address to the ICN, Fenwick inaugurated the custom of providing a watchword for each 5-year period of the ICN's work. This speech also gave Fenwick her first opportunity publicly to expound on the ICN's mission.

> The organization of the International Council is as simple as it is sure. The graduate nurses combine to form Alumnae Associations; by delegation these societies cooperate to form a National Association. The National Associated Alumnae in conjunction with the Superintendents' Society, federate to make a National Council, and the National Councils are then eligible for affiliation with the International Council of Nurses.

In this fashion, Fenwick concluded, the ICN would secure for each graduate member a voice in her professional affairs, or what she termed *professional suffrage*.[38]

At the same time she called for unity, Fenwick also stressed the need for accommodating diversity. "In a society which would be worldwide, which would include members of every race and creed, we must, while maintaining inviolate certain broad general principles which form our common bond of union, permit—nay foster—individuality in detail, authorizing each country to apply these principles in a manner best suited to its own needs," she argued.[39]

In practical terms, Fenwick directed the members' energies to the creation of the national councils. She urged that in the process of forming the councils, nursing leaders allow for individuality. "Diversity of opinion is the very salt of life, and we shall do well to encourage rather than deprecate its expression," she suggested. After Fenwick's address, the assembled group heard progress reports on nursing organization in various countries. Both first-hand accounts and written summaries described conditions in Australia, Brazil, Canada, Cuba, Denmark, Egypt, France, Great Britain and Ireland, Holland, Italy, New Zealand, Norway, South Africa, and the United States.

At the end of its deliberations, the ICN decided to meet again in Berlin in 1904. The members then adjourned to join in the Third International Nursing Congress, at which many of them gave papers: Ethel Gordon Fenwick on "A Plea for Higher Education of Nurses," Mary Agnes Snively on "Organization and Legislation Among Nurses in Canada," Isla Stewart on "Hospital Administration in Great Britain," Sarah McGahey on the "Nurses' Federation of Australia," and Lavinia Dock on "What Are We Doing With the Three Years' Course?" In these speeches before the Congress, leaders of the early ICN elaborated on the program for nursing uplift they envisioned in their own countries.

Even more revealing of the newly formed ICN agenda were the informal reports on the status of nursing presented at the Buffalo Congress. These reports, which were later published as part of the ICN proceedings, provide a fascinating survey of world nursing, as seen through the eyes of Anglo-American nurses. Fenwick apparently used her personal network to solicit the reports, so even in countries such as Brazil, Egypt, or France where British nurses were by no means representative of the dominant nursing tradition, it was they who were asked to provide their impressions. The end result was a highly ethnocentric survey of the nursing world. Two tendencies characteristic of the Anglo-American nursing tradition were the negative characterizations of the European Catholic countries and the missionary overtones of the reports on nursing in Britain's overseas colonies.

The report presented on France by Dr. Anna Hamilton was thought to be so important that it was read in full. Anna Hamilton had recently taken charge of a hospital training school in Bordeaux and was setting it "on a proper footing for lady probationers," with "properly trained nurses to instruct them." Her report on French nursing began with an extended and devastating critique of the Roman Catholic nursing orders that held an exclusive monopoly on hospital nursing until the late 1870s.

When reform sprung up in Protestant countries, it was not taken into consideration by the religious bodies who ruled the hospitals through the

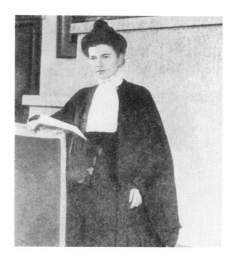

**FIGURE 1-7**
*Anna Hamilton reading her thesis on nursing at Montpellier. From LL Dock, History of Nursing, Vol. 3, 1912.*

nuns, and these last, kept aloof from all that goes on in the world, went on exactly in their work as they were wont to do ages ago.

Specifically, Hamilton criticized nuns' lack of formal nursing training and inability to work at night, attend male patients, help women in child-birth, give vaginal douches, or administer enemas. "Their lay helpers, ignorant and worse, and the medical students do what proper nurses would accomplish ever so much better, being refined and womanly." In 1877, the municipal council of Paris decided to start secular schools for the sick, but in Hamilton's words, "this assembly of men, though clever enough and lovers of progress, did not understand at all the requisites for securing proper training for nurses." The municipal schools quickly degenerated into diploma mills, where there was little integration of theoretical and practical work. If one had any doubts about how poorly the new schools were serving their purpose, Hamilton concluded, "the actual state of Paris hospitals proves it at one glance."[40]

Amy Turton's account of nursing in Italy, which was also read in full, was only slightly less critical. She too described the lack of training common among the religious nursing orders and the important nursing tasks left to their lay servants. She described the first training school, established in Rome in 1892 or 1893, as a good-intentioned but flawed effort at reform. Turton noted, "Italians have great facility for grasping most things, and these girls learned well everything that was taught." But, she continued, "The misfortune was that so many things were not taught at all, and others were mistaught." The hospital had no matron, so a surgeon and his assistants provided instruction to the nursing students. "The ethics of nursing thus became falsified, and the girls refused to do the humbler offices for the sick," calling for servants to perform them or simply leaving them undone.[41]

In contrast, Lavinia Dock's report on German nursing stressed the high achievements of the Protestant nursing orders, which through the example of Kaiserswerth had so influenced the work of Florence Nightingale. "It is from the German forms that the English and our own nursing systems have developed," she noted. She praised not only the deaconess tradition, but the newer, secular nursing associations established in Berlin and Hamburg. But Dock found disturbing what she saw as the lack of autonomy among German nurses and their leaders. Even the efforts to give nurses more autonomy, she noted, were initiated by "pastors of 'liberal views,' and all textbooks, lectures to nurses, histories of nursing, theories of nursing and rules of conduct for nurses, are written by men."

Dock continued, "An American is astonished at the silence among these women of the Old World." She noted with dismay that "the superintendents of nurses in these vast establishments, women of immense ability and possessing authority in certain directions more extensive than any of our superintendents possess, have no associate life." Some German nurses longed for more independence, but their lot, Dock observed, was a sad one. "One longs to help them but does not know how." They must help themselves, she concluded, and change will "be the result of a long, slow process."[42]

Although also finding much to criticize, the ICN progress reports on nursing in the colonies were curiously more forgiving of local lapses. Anna Hamilton found the untrained nurses and embedded dirt in the hospitals of France, a supposedly civilized nation, far more contemptible than did her contemporaries confronting similar problems in Fiji or Zanzibar. Colonialist assumptions about the responsibility of English-trained nurses to uplift the natives and the ingrained limits of the latter's abilities softened nurses' accounts of deficiencies found in non-Western countries.

The English-trained nurses' reports on these countries stayed in the mode of missionary accounts. They saw themselves as representing not only nursing, but also English civilization. Their commentaries suggested that English ways would come only slowly to native cultures, but they expressed a strong sense of optimism that their civilizing influence was all to the good.

May Anderson's observations on "Nursing in Fiji" conveyed the patient, maternalistic tone common to these reports. She described the island's hospital, begun in 1883 "by erecting a few native houses of unsawn timber, reeds and thatch: not aseptic, perhaps, many nurses may think, and quite correctly so, yet for a time they served their purpose in sheltering patients who came from neighboring or distant islands." The hospital was originally under the care of an "untrained matron who was kind, indeed to the patients, but lacked the knowledge so essential in nursing the sick." The colonial governor realized that further improvement was needed, so a proper English nurse trained at St. Thomas's Hospital in London came to replace her. That matron began to train native women as probationers, who after graduation were sent to nurse in the provinces under the direction of the local medical officer. This tradition of bringing "old-time probationers" over from England to keep the hospital and training school in order had continued to the present day.[43]

As did many of the English nurses providing the ICN with reports, Anderson included many observations on the racial traits of the natives. "As with all uncultured people," she remarked, "the Fijians have curious ideas about soap and water, and when not under European supervision they allow their sick to lie for weeks and even months and never dream of washing or sponging them, or even combing their thick hair." She noted that patient diets could be a difficulty: "as we try to give to each according to their religious and caste prejudices, the diet list often presents a very complicated bill of fare." Local racial prejudices shaped the plan of the hospital. It was just as well the buildings did not conform to the desired pavilion plan she noted, because having many individual wards made it easier to keep separate the Europeans, Fijians, Indian coolies and "strays" from other nations. "The Europeans' wards are fitted with all the ordinary ward furniture, and are very bright and cheerful," observed Anderson. "The native wards are not supplied with more than is really necessary, as native habits are usually somewhat grimy and disagreeable, and nurses must ever be on the alert to keep everything clean."[44]

Lucy W. Quintard's report on Cuba confirms that the missionary stance was not limited to the English nurses. Compared to its European counterparts, the United States came late and more uneasily to imperialism, only acquiring its first colonial possessions in 1898, after the Spanish-American War. Quintard's account of nursing reform under the American occupation of Cuba resembled in many respects the British nurses' colonial narratives. The hospitals under the old regime were "dens of immorality and uncleanliness in every form." Nursing was the province of untrained men and women, "the lowest type of humanity." She believed that the term *enfermero*, or *nurse*, was a term of insult.

> Recognizing the herculean task before them of cleaning up these hospitals, and realizing their helplessness to accomplish it singlehanded, the men to whom this work was entrusted turned to the nursing profession for assistance, and they met with a hearty response.[45]

Well-qualified graduate nurses from American schools went to the island to set up training schools at the largest hospitals.

Quintard compared their task to the early history of the American hospital schools. As she pointed out, in both instances, strong prejudices against both hospitals and work for women outside the home had to be conquered. Although praising the Cuban women for their intelligence and quickness, Quintard noted that they had certain weaknesses stemming from years of Spanish rule. A "Cuban girl thinks no more of telling a falsehood than the truth," she claimed, because of the long necessity of shielding friends and relatives from the imperial foes. "Time and training are the only remedies, and on these two factors we must depend for improvement." In conclusion, Quintard appealed to her "northern" colleagues to help in Cuban work. "Never could one undertake better missionary work than in devoting a couple of years to one of our Cuba schools."[46]

## The Berlin Congress, 1904

The next meeting of the ICN, which was held in Berlin in conjunction with the International Congress of Women, turned the spotlight of criticism on the situation in German nursing. The prospect of visiting Germany inspired a special sense of excitement and reflection among the ICN leaders. As an editorial in the *British Journal of Nursing* (BJN) observed,

> [N]o English nurse can set foot on German soil without remembering with a thrill that she is in the country which gave Frederica Fliedner to the world. That at Kaiserswerth, on the Rhine, was evolved, under her control, the system of nursing which sent Florence Nightingale, trained and disciplined, to wrestle triumphantly with the disorganization of hospital management in the Crimea, and subsequently to found in this country, for the first time on a scientific basis, a training school for nurses in connection with St. Thomas's Hospital.

What, then, could English nurses give their German sisters in return, the editorial asked rhetorically?[47] As various articles by English and American nursing leaders made evident, the answer to that question was to help them reform themselves in the image of Anglo-American nurses.

Dock had already made clear in her report at the Buffalo meeting that the ICN leadership believed the continued dominance of the religious sisterhoods stifled German nursing. Despite the high level of their technical ability, nurses there lacked the opportunity to think and act for themselves. The BJN editorial concluded of the upcoming meeting, "It were happiness indeed if we could set their feet in the way of professional independence—independence both of thought and action." In practical terms, this meant supporting the growth of the Free Sisterhood, that is, the organization of nurses independent of the religious orders.[48]

## Nursing in Germany

Certainly, nursing emerged in turmoil during the late 19th century in Germany. Strikes of dissatisfied deaconess nurses and sisters of the Order of St. John in some of the hospitals in Hamburg attracted public attention.[49] Not only was inappropriate care in the hospitals widely discussed in the newspapers, but influential physicians, members of parliament, and practicing nurses began to question the lack of legal regulations and proper education for nurses. Some accused nurses of being uncivilized and uneducated, whereas others argued that nurses were victims of exploitation and inappropriate labor conditions.[50]

The publication of *"Die Soziale Stellung der Krankenpflegerinnen"* [The social position of nurses] by Elisabeth Storp, a nurse trained in the Victoria House in Berlin, provoked the public debate. In it, Storp discussed the working conditions and exploitation of German nurses, and compared the wages of nurses with those of teachers. Storp challenged nurses to establish a committee to advocate for state-approved education and legal protection of nurses' work.[51] What Lavinia Dock called the "revolt against unpaid labor of women" was a significant element in nursing's transition from a charitable and religious enterprise to a paid professional occupation.[52]

Most nursing of the sick in 19th-century Germany was done by Catholic and Protestant groups of religious women. The most famous deaconess institute was Kaiserswerth, established by Pastor Fliedner in 1836, which so impressed Florence Nightingale.[53] By 1850, Fliedner's Institute consisted of "a hospital nursing school, a motherhouse (for nurses and teachers), an orphanage, a teacher's seminary for infant, elementary and industrial schoolteachers, an infant school and an asylum for the female mentally ill.[54]

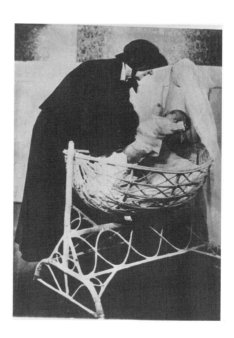

**FIGURE 1-8**
*A Protestant Deaconess—early 20th century. From Lynaugh Collection, Bryn Mawr, PA.*

Catholic sisters and Protestant deaconesses were organized in mother-houses where women from respectable families could pursue a socially accepted public role. Devoting themselves to works of charity, they were bound to the motherhouse for life. In exchange for their work, they received shelter, food, clothing, pocket money and provision for old age.[55] They did not receive any personal salary. The motherhouse was strictly hierarchical; sisters could be sent wherever the head of the house ordered them to go. Nurse training in the motherhouses was grounded in the principles of order, discipline and obedience, and generally contained some medical instruction.[56] Pastor Fliedner, in particular, designed a detailed rule of conduct for his deaconess sisterhood to ensure that nursing be seen as an acceptable career for middle-class women. The motherhouse system was such a powerful model that patriotic associations for the care of wounded soldiers, established during the 19th century and eventually merging to become the Red Cross, adopted much of the motherhouse idea.[57]

Begun as a nursing reform in the early 1800s, the motherhouse system seemed too rigid and inflexible by the end of the 19th century. This was particularly true in the light of the demands of a new generation of women. In the rapidly growing cities, many nurses separated themselves from the motherhouses and began to work either in private duty or in the municipal hospitals. Women's changing role in society, a growing women's movement, and the need for women to make a living increased the view among many nurses that the motherhouses were too restrictive. As was true of women around the world, a new generation of German nurses sought economic independence and a more autonomous life.[58]

Nevertheless, the free or wild nurses, as those who had separated themselves from motherhouses were called, were still vulnerable, risking their reputations and remaining largely unprotected and isolated.[59] Paid nursing service was a way to earn a living, but work conditions, especially in the urban hospitals, were harsh. Lack of legal protection or regulation of training for nurses made independent nurses prone to exploitation. With help from charity and endowments, motherhouses offered nursing at prices far lower than those required by independent nurses. In this competition with motherhouses, independent nurses found low wages and poor working conditions. Nurses were not covered by state social security laws for sickness, disability and old age. Many experienced poor physical and mental health at early ages.[60]

## Agnes Karll

It was this situation that Agnes Karll sought to change when she founded the Professional Organization for German Nurses in 1903 (*Berufsorganisation der Krankenpflegerinnen Deutschlands*). Agnes Karll, born in 1868,

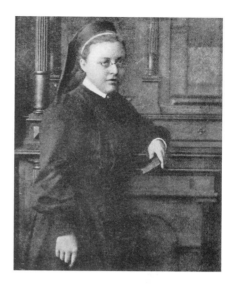

**FIGURE 1-9**

*Agnes Karll, Founder of the German Nurses Association and ICN President, 1909 to 1912. From LL Dock, History of Nursing, Vol. 4, 1912.*

daughter of an estate owner, initially attended a preparatory school for teachers but then, at age 19, entered nurse training at the Clementinen House in Hannover, a Red Cross motherhouse.[61] Family obligations forced Karll into independent work, and she did private duty in Berlin from 1891 to 1901.[62] Although her patients were primarily from higher social classes referred from well-educated family doctors, the hard work still led to her physical breakdown at age 33.

When her health forced her to abandon private duty, Karll turned to the betterment of nurses' social conditions. Her own personal experiences increased her understanding of the needs of nurses. Karll did not yet have a clear idea of how she would pursue her goal of nursing improvement, but she used her connections with the women's movement and her knowledge about insurance for nurses to develop her ideas. She looked into state and private insurance opportunities for nurses, searching for solutions so nurses could protect themselves financially against the risk of old age and invalidity.[63] Karll knew Adele Schreiber, who was employed by a private insurance company, the *Deutsche Anker,* to look after the insurance needs of a growing group of employed women.[64] Because nurses were exempted from the compulsory social insurance established for laborers in late 19th-century Germany, Schreiber helped Karll envision a program of private insurance for nurses. As a result of this relationship, Karll became the first nurse insured with the *Deutsche Anker.*

Karll was also influenced by the writings of Elisabeth Storp and Marie Cauer. Cauer, a nurse writing about the condition of nurses, was the step-daughter of a leading figure in the German Women's Association (GWA).[65] During the summer of 1902, Karll met with Storp, Cauer, and

Cauer's associate, Helene Meyer, in Berlin. The nurses' difficult professional plight attracted the attention of the GWA through Storp's writings. The GWA leaders accepted a paper on nursing at the 1902 national meeting of the association in Wiesbaden, which Cauer, Karll, Storp, and Meyer were invited to prepare and present. Initially, Karll hesitated because her primary interest lay in improving the situation of independent private-duty nurses. The GWA was more concerned with changing the training and working conditions for hospital-based nurses through licensing and state registration. Gradually, however, she began to see the need for nursing organization and the improvement of education and legal regulation as complementary strategies to achieve nurses' social improvement.

The Wiesbaden meeting was Karll's first public event. The *Deutsche Anker* insurance company paid for her travel expenses.[66] Meeting with 230 other women, Karll was immediately caught up in the excitement of great gatherings of women. During the meeting, she made valuable contacts; she was encouraged to create an organization of nurses. All this convinced Karll that such an organization was imperative if nurses were to become independent.

Back in Berlin, Karll set about creating her organization. She gathered a group of seven nurses in a preparatory committee for the foundation of an independent Professional Organization of German Nurses (POGN). After studying American examples, Karll designed a draft of the association's bylaws with Maria Cauer's assistance.[67] The association's objective was to actively mediate private-duty nurses' placement through an employment bureau, and its bylaws also required that members of the organization seek personal financial protection through insurance.[68] The founding meeting, on January 11, 1903, attracted about 30 nurses. These first members of the organization elected the preparatory committee as the board of directors, and Agnes Karll as the association president.

As most were unfamiliar with leadership responsibilities, they hesitated to take on secretarial and managerial tasks. Karll noted, "None of us had ever taken minutes, not to mention having ever chaired a meeting."[69] Karll and her colleagues spent all their spare time and energy on creating the POGN and the nursing bureau. To be recognized as a legal body, the association obtained corporation rights from local government officials. Bylaws were printed and sent to 2400 physicians in Berlin and suburbs. Initially, the bureau hired just one paid worker; within a year, however, they attracted 300 members. During the first 5 years, the bureau grew to a busy office with about 10 paid workers. In a few more years, the POGN stood as a flourishing organization of over 3000 members. An extensive network of nurses throughout the country with local subdivisions was established, headed by a nurse if at all possible. Karll traveled extensively, speaking to nurses, city officials, women, and physicians about the new idea of an independent nursing association. The POGN established its own journal in 1905, for which Karll wrote most of the editorials.

The independent POGN's relationship with the motherhouses was tense. When POGN chose the Lazarus Cross as its badge, a sign once carried by a knightly order during the crusades, the Red Cross motherhouses complained that the symbol was too close to that of the Red Cross. The lawsuit the Red Cross initiated was, however, won by the POGN.[70] During their first public meeting, POGN nurses were challenged by some influential physicians for calling themselves "sisters." The use of this title of public respect for the work of the nurse was defended by one of the POGN board members. She argued that independent professional nurses were, indeed, forming a unified sisterhood.[71]

Karll actively mediated the placement of nurses either in hospitals or private-duty positions. One of her main concerns was the poor health and relatively high suicide rate among nurses. In a letter to Lavinia Dock, Karll wrote, "Saturday I have to go to a little town one hour distant to look after one of our sisters, who tried to take her life, because she feels, she will not very long be able to work. It is heart rending."[72]

Through her connections to the international women's movement, Karll attracted the attention of nurses forming the ICN. In 1904, when the ICN gathered at the meeting of the ICW in Berlin, she was invited to speak, and the POGN was admitted as a founding member. But, at the same time, resistance to Karll's ideas among German nurses became evident during the discussion at the Nursing Section. Frau Thusnelda Arndt, representing one of the Red Cross sisterhoods, spoke out sharply against the Free Sisterhood movement on the grounds that "the nursing profession was not, and must not be, a business to get money by." She insisted that nurses had to be dedicated to humanity, not to making a living. "Only an organized sisterhood could give a nurse the standing which she needed; she could never attain it in a society founded on a pecuniary basis."[73]

Isla Stewart responded to Arndt with a speech that summed up the general principles of the ICN. She stated unequivocally that "the right of nurses to absolute freedom, after their training was complete, to take up any branch of work which they desired, and to determine the conditions under which they would work, were points which could not be too strongly insisted upon." These were the conditions that had allowed American and English nurses to better themselves, she insisted. The key to nursing progress lay in creating associations of certified nurses and achieving state registration.[74]

Karll envied the accomplishments of American and English colleagues and perceived the unity of the American and English nursing organizations to be in great contrast to the narrow-minded "caste" mentality of the German nursing leaders.[75] She maintained a regular correspondence with Lavinia Dock, with whom she shared both her hopes and frustration about German nursing developments.[76] The state-regulated, 3-year nurse training model that Karll promoted accorded with ICN standards. The eventual outcome of the German political battle over nursing education, however, disappointed her. The Prussian state government proposed to give a state examination after only 1 year of nurses' training. This recommendation became effective in Prussia in 1907, and soon after that in many other states.[77] Although Karll saw the law as an important first step, she was frustrated that nurses had little, if any, control over the examination, its content, or the judging of examinees; all this was reserved to physicians.

## The Business of the Berlin Meeting

By 1904, the first quinquennial of the ICN, three nations, Germany, Great Britain, and the United States, had formed national councils and were ready for federation. The meeting in Berlin, held at the Victoria Lyceum on June 17, was attended by a much larger contingent of delegates than the previous one: 30 nurses came from England, Scotland, and Ireland; 28 from the United States; 24 from Germany; and there were individual representatives from Australia, Canada, Sweden, and France.

In the morning session, the assembled group received from Fenwick the watchword for the next quinquennial—courage—and heard progress reports on the development of national councils in the United States, England, Germany, and Ireland. In recognition of the longstanding difficulties over Ireland, the minutes record that "the President thought the Irish Nurses Association might prefer entering as a national body by itself, and not as included in the English National Committee." In other business, the ICN decided to use the *British Journal of Nursing* and the *American Journal of Nursing* as their official organs. The body elected new officers: Susan B. McGahey of Australia became the new president, Lavinia Dock

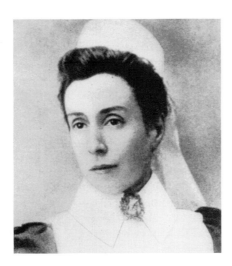

**FIGURE 1-10**
*Susan B. McGahey of Australia, ICN President 1904 to 1909. LL Dock, A History of Nursing, Vol. 4, 1912.*

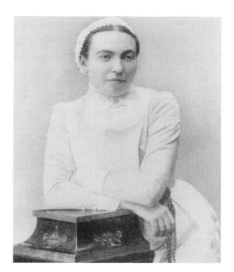

**FIGURE 1-11**
*Margaret Breay, Honorary Treasurer
of ICN for 21 years. From LL Dock,
History of Nursing, Vol. 3, 1912.*

continued as secretary, and England's Margaret Breay became the new treasurer.[78]

In the afternoon session, the delegates heard invited papers on the state of nursing legislation in England, the United States, New Zealand, and Australia, followed by a paper on nursing education submitted by Adelaide Nutting of the United States. The latter provoked an extended discussion, after which Fenwick proposed a series of resolutions that concisely summed up the ICN's program for nursing reform.

Fenwick began with a series of propositions laying the groundwork for the standards to be enacted. The first resolution stated that "the disorder existing today in nursing conditions is due chiefly to inequalities of training and differing educational standards." The second stipulated that "the serious and responsible work of a nurse demands not only excellent moral qualities but also the trained intelligence and cultured mind of the well-educated woman." The third proposition held that "the principle of Registration by the state is now generally conceded as safeguarding the public health, and as promoting a more thorough education of nurses."[79]

Holding these propositions to be true, the ICN established the following minimum criteria for the trained nurse: "a good general education"; a preliminary course covering "domestic science, elementary anatomy, physiology, bacteriology, materia medica, and technical preparation for ward work"; and 3 years of "practical work in hospital wards under qualified instructors." The final resolutions dealt with the certification of these accomplishments arguing that the state should provide a system for examining and registering trained nurses who met stipulated criteria. In addition, "it is the duty of the Training Schools to certify to the qualities of character and moral fitness of candidates for registration." The education agenda was passed unanimously, and the meeting was concluded.[80]

## The "Four Lions" and Unity

The community of nurses envisioned by the early leaders of the ICN was strongly shaped by the missionary and suffragist elements of the larger 19th-century women's movement. Fenwick, Dock, and their fellow nurses thought of themselves as apostles of a new nursing sisterhood, formed in the image of the Anglo-American nursing movement, with its more secular, professional orientation, and its strong commitment to women's rights. Promoting those goals among the nurses of all lands was the ultimate goal of their ICN, as they conceived it.

Although the Anglo-American leadership of the ICN shared similar beliefs about women's proper role in society and the superiority of their own culture, they also perceived among themselves a clear division between the Old World and the New. By virtue of their youth, the United States, New Zealand, and Australia were seen as more progressive in the areas of both nursing and women's rights than their mother country of England, which, in turn, was seen as more liberal than the nations of continental Europe. By bringing the Old World and the New together, the ICN would act as a force against professional backwardness.

Lavinia Dock summarized the ICN's mission for the ASSTSN in 1905. Here, she most clearly spells out her vision of the organization's missionary role. To give her American colleagues some sense of their special duties in the ICN, she gave them an overview, based on her travels and researches, of "the difficulties of our foreign sisters." She began by reminding them that "whereas we in America have only an educational problem, that is a single-faced problem, the pioneers of modern Nursing in Europe have a four-fold opposition to overcome." The "four lions" that European nurses faced were, according to Dock, religious, social, masculine, and industrial prejudice.[81]

First, in many European nations, it required a bitter struggle to "secure the right of nursing to be 'unconfessional' or independent of religious orders." Dock reminded her listeners that the struggle involved not just "lofty spiritual domination" but the financial control of nurses as well. Second, Dock thought the greater class distinctions present in European society heightened the division between classes of nurses; those of higher social classes dominated administration, whereas those from the peasant and servant classes did the difficult manual labor. This class issue posed a "dead weight" on efforts at educational reform and nursing self-governance. Dock also noted that class prejudice hurt women who became nurses to support themselves because it was not considered respectable to work for money.[82]

As for masculine prejudice, Dock said she did not need to elaborate. "I would only like to say that in no country of the world, unless perhaps New Zealand and Australia, are men in general so fair to women, and the medical profession in particular so generous and so brotherly towards nurses, as in America." Obviously expecting that some in her audience might find this confident comparison hard to accept, Dock assured them that exceptions to her generalization about masculine benevolence were "insignificant." She stated flatly, "I have made many scientific investigations upon this subject and I have collected much valuable data."[83]

Dock's final "lion" was the problem of industrial prejudice or what she said might be better termed *industrial superstition*. Referring particularly to the situation in England, she observed how the comparison between the nursing registration movement and the trades union movement was used to denigrate the former. Such claims, Dock asserted, reflected a "sordid fear of allowing nurses to work for reforms through their own associations."[84]

"These four lions lie in the path of our over-seas sisters," Dock concluded. "In one country one will be found more prominent, in another, another, but in every country they are all present to some extent and in varying proportions." She then went on in a country-by-country account making explicit her bedrock assumption that the only good nursing associations were those entirely controlled by nurses, and entirely independent of religious orders.[85]

As Diane Hamilton has shown in her analysis of the mind of nursing at the turn of the century, Lavinia Dock and her fellow "nurse inventors" were intent upon severing professional nursing from its roots in the nursing sisterhoods. Hamilton writes, "To these nurse inventors, the church's requirement of blind obedience negated emancipation for womanhood, diminished the hope of a better life for humans, and threatened [their] ideal of nursing having a voice of its own."[86] Dock's uneasiness with the religious orders reflected no disregard for the spiritual dignity of nursing, which she believed in wholeheartedly. Her ideal of nursing compassion had deep roots in 19th-century Protestantism. Rather, for Dock, the more pressing problem was female *autonomy*. Where nurses had to speak through any sort of a hierarchy, particularly one dominated by men, they had no voice of their own.

In Dock's conception, then, the New World nurses' participation in the ICN was a form of missionary work bound up in ideals of compassion and female autonomy. This American agenda was bound to cause tensions for the ICN as it tried to build outward from its original core of Anglo-American members. As we have seen, in countries such as France and Germany, Dock's requirements for secularization and female autonomy posed serious barriers to enlisting widespread nursing participation.

Less obviously troublesome to Dock and the other founders, but equally problematic in the long run, was the missionary mind they shared with other members of their class. The ICN incorporated, almost unconsciously, the shape of the colonial world as it existed in the decades preceding World War I. No more and no less than their male contemporaries, these women held assumptions about the superiority of Anglo-American political institutions and social forms, a superiority that was rooted in race as well as culture. Their maternalistic standards for nursing in nonwhite countries implicitly took white, Western European culture as the yardstick for progress. Only after that political world began to crumble would those basic assumptions about empire and racial superiority be exposed and put to the test.

## ENDNOTES

1. Bridges, *A History*, 7–8.
2. Nancy Cott, *The Grounding of Modern Feminism* (New Haven, CT: Yale University Press, 1987), 3. For general accounts of the origins of the women's movement, see Jane Rendall, *The Origins of Modern Feminism: Women in Britain, France, and the United States, 1780–1860* (New York: Schocken Books, 1984); Richard J. Evans, *The Feminists* (London: Croom Helm, 1977); and Anne Firor Scott, *Natural Allies: Women's Associations in American History* (Chicago: University of Illinois Press, 1993).
3. Janet Saltzman Chafetz, Anthony Gary Dworkin, and Stephanie Swanson, "Social Changes and Social Activism: First-Wave Women's Movements Around the World," in Guida West and Rhoda Lois Blumberg, Eds., *Women and Social Protest* (New York: Oxford University Press, 1990), 302–320. The authors note that independent women's movements were largely a middle-class urban phenomenon.
4. Jane Hunter, *The Gospel of Gentility: American Women Missionaries in Turn-of-the-Century China* (New Haven, CT: Yale University Press, 1984) quoting from Beecher's *Treatise on Domestic Economy* (1842).
5. Thomas Dublin, *Women at Work: The Transformation of Work and Community in Lowell, Massachusetts, 1826–1869* (New York: Columbia University Press, 1979).
6. Peggy Pascoe, *Relations of Rescue: The Search for Female Moral Authority in the American West, 1874–1939* (New York and Oxford: Oxford University Press, 1990).
7. Hunter, *The Gospel of Gentility*, 1984, xx.
8. Hunter, *The Gospel of Gentility*, xiii. Joan Jacobs Brumberg, *Mission for Life* (New York: The Free Press, 1980), recounts the enormous interest in Judson and his three wives.
9. Patricia R. Hill, *The World Their Household: The American Woman's Foreign Mission Movement and Cultural Transformation, 1870–1920* (Ann Arbor, MI: The University of Michigan Press, 1984). Hill examines the cultural and ideological climate that made foreign missions an especially congenial object for female benevolence in the years immediately following the Civil War.
10. Joan Jacobs Brumberg, "Zenanas and Girlless Villages: An Ethnology of American Evangelical Women, 1870–1910," *Journal of American History*, 69 (September 1982): 347–371, suggests how evangelical women constructed a sense of comradeship with "heathen women" that reinforced their own sense of racial and cultural superiority. For imagined community, see Benedict Anderson, *Imagined Communities: Reflections on the Origin and Spread of Nationalism* (London and New York: Verso, 1991). We have

found Anderson's exploration of the personal and cultural implications of belonging to a nation helpful in considering the historical meaning of the ICN.

11. Ellen Carol DuBois, *Feminism and Suffrage: The Emergence of an Independent Women's Movement in America, 1848–1869* (Ithaca: Cornell University Press, 1978; on British women and antislavery, see Claire Midgeley, *Women Against Slavery: The British Campaigns, 1780–1830* (New York: Routledge, 1994).

12. For general accounts of the women's suffrage movement, see Susan Kingsley Kent, *Sex and Suffrage in Britain, 1860–1914* (Princeton: Princeton University Press, 1987). Sources give three different dates for the founding of the National Society: 1867, 1868, and 1869.

13. Brumberg, "Zenanas," 351.

14. Ian Tyrrell, *Women's World, Women's Empire: The Woman's Christian Temperance Union in International Perspective, 1880–1930* (Chapel Hill and London: The University of North Carolina Press, 1991).

15. Wendy Mitchinson, "The Woman's Christian Temperance Union: A Study in Organization," *International Journal of Women's Studies*, 4 (March/April 1981): 143–156.

16. This history of the ICW is drawn from International Council of Women, *Women in a Changing World: The Dynamic Story of the International Council of Women Since 1888* (London: Routledge & Kegan Paul, 1966). On the internationalizing impulse in the women's suffrage movement, see Caroline Daley and Melanie Nolan, *Suffrage and Beyond: International Feminist Perspectives* (New York: New York University Press, 1994).

17. Ibid., quotation on 15.

18. Stanton's speech is reprinted in "Formal Opening of the Council," *Report of the International Council of Women, Assembled by the National Woman Suffrage Association . . . 1888* (Washington, DC: Rufus Darby, Printer, 1888), 31–39; quotations are from 33.

19. Preamble of ICW constitution, quoted in Bridges, *A History*, 2–3.

20. International Council of Women, *Women in a Changing World*, circular quoted on 17. See Diane Hamilton, "Earnest Thought: The Columbian Exposition, 1893," American Association for the History of Nursing Annual Meeting, 1993, on the significance of the 1893 exposition for the nursing profession.

21. Quoted in Virginia Arnold, "The Past: The Way to the Future," *International Nursing Review*, 21:3–4 (1974): 69.

22. On the politics of the registration movement, see Nancy Tomes, "The Silent Battle: Nurse Registration in New York State, 1903–20," in *Nursing History: New Perspectives, New Possibilities*, Ellen Lagemann, Ed. (New York: Teachers College Press, 1983), 107–132.

23. Ethel Fenwick, "Nursing At the World's Fair," *Nursing Record* (January 26, 1893): 52–59; quotations are on 54 and 53.

24. [Grace] Neill, "The Professional Training and Status of Nurses," in International Congress of Women, *Women in Professions, Being the Professional Section of the International Congress of Women, London, July, 1899*, 2 vols. (London: T. Fisher Unwin, 1900), vol. 2, 3–8; quotation is on 8.

25. M. H. Watkins, "State Registration of Nurses at Cape Colony, in *Women in Professions*, vol. 2, 8–11; quotation is on 10.

26. [Isabel] Hampton Robb, "The Organization of Trained Nurses' Alumnae Associations," in *Women in Professions*, vol. 2, 28–33; quotation is on 29.

27. Neill, "The Professional Training," 6.

28. Lavinia Dock, "Discussion of State Registration for Nurses," in *Women in Professions*, vol. 2, 11–13; quotation is on 13.

29. Mary Agnes Snively, "Discussion of Trained Nurses Alumnae Associations," in *Women in Professions*, vol. 2, 33–34; quotation is on 33.

30. "Nursing at the International Congress," *Nursing Record* (May 20, 1899): 397–398; quotation is on 398.

31. Lavinia Dock, "The International Council of Nurses," *American Journal of Nursing*, 1 (October, 1900): 114.

32. Text from clipping in front of ICN Minute Book, 1899–1904, Book 2. ICNA.

33. ICN Minutes, 1899–1904, Book 1, 6. ICNA.

34. A clipping pasted in ICN Minutes, 1899–1904, Book 2, contains the text of Sewall's speech.

35. For discussion of the Constitution, and the agreed upon draft, see ICN Minutes, 1899–1904, Book 1, pp 7–27. ICNA.

36. Quoted in Bridges, *A History*, 230.

37. ICN Minutes, 1899–1904, Book 1, pp 19–20.

38. "Address of the President" [Ethel Gordon Fenwick], in *Transactions of the Third International Congress of Nurses, With Reports of the International Council of Nurses, Buffalo, 1901* [hereafter ICN Reports 1901] 379–383; quotation is on 381.

39. Ibid., 381–382.

40. Anna Hamilton, "Nursing in France," ICN Reports 1901, 417–423, quotations are on 418, 419, 421.

41. Amy Turton, "Nursing in Italy," ICN Reports 1901, 464–469; quotation is on 464.

42. Lavinia Dock, "Nursing Organization in Germany," ICN Reports 1901, 443–451; quotations are on 448–449.

43. May Anderson, "Nursing in Fiji," ICN Reports 1901, 410–416; quotations are on 410, 411.

44. Ibid., 412, 413.

45. Lucy W. Quintard, "Nursing in Cuba," ICN Reports 1901, 396–401; quotation is on 396.

46. Ibid., 399, 400.

47. Editorial, "At Berlin," *British Journal of Nursing*, 32 (May 21, 1904).

48. Ibid.

49. *Trained Nurse and Hospital Review*, LXXII, 223; Agnes Karll, *History of the First Five Years of Our Association* (Berlin: Deutscher Verlag, 1908), 1. This section on Germany relies importantly on Geertje Boschma, "Reviews of Selected Histories on Belgium, France, Germany, Holland and Great Britain," unpublished manuscript, University of Pennsylvania, 1993.

50. A. P. Kruse, *Nursing Education Since the Mid-19th Century* (Stuttgart: Kohlhammer, 1987), 69–105.

51. M. Lungershausen, *Agnes Karll, Her Life, Works and Inheritance* (Hannover: Elwin Staude Verlag, 1964), 13–17; Agnes Karll, 1908, 1.

52. Quotation is from Lavinia Dock, *A History of Nursing, Volume IV* (New York: Putnam, 1912), 7, who described the efforts of independent nurses in Germany to establish themselves as respected paid professionals breaking with the traditional congregational nursing system.

53. Kruse, 1987, 38–39.

54. Irene Poplin, *A Study of the Kaiserswerth Deaconess Institutes' Nurse Training School in 1850–51: Purpose and Curriculum* (The University of Texas at Austin: PhD Dissertation, 1988), 40.

55. Dock, 1912, 4–5.
56. Poplin, 1988, 53–57, 276–317.
57. Kruse, 1987, 43–51. For a discussion of institutions and organizations that served as alternative families for 19th century women in Great Britain, see Martha Vicinus, *Independent Women: Work and Community for Single Women, 1850–1920* (Chicago and London: University of Chicago Press, 1985).
58. During the 19th century, liberal and later socialist movements developed in Germany. Within this context, the women's movement grew, advocating for women's suffrage and fighting for economic independence for women. This provided a context for nurses to improve their situation as Agnes Karll strove to do. For a discussion, see Lungershausen, *Agnes Karll, Her Life, Work and Inheritance*. (Hannover: Elvin Staude Verlag, 1964).
59. Lungershausen (1964) defines the 'free or wild nurses' (pp 13–14) as the growing group of nurses who provided care without any affiliation to a motherhouse, found especially in the large cities. These included women who started as ward attendants and those who separated themselves from one of the motherhouses and worked independently. What was controversial about this group was that they worked for a living and were without legal protection.
60. Claudia Bischoff, *Frauen in der Krankenpflege: Zur Entwichlung von Frauenrolle und Frauenberufstatigheit in 19 und 20 Jahrhundert* (Frankfurtamain: Campus Verlag, 1984), 94–103, 108–109. Bischoff argues that the unprotected status of the independent nurses forced them into long hours, often working through the night and with rare days off.
61. The head of the school, Johanna Wilborn, described by Karll as an advocate of women's emancipation and self-organization of teachers, developed a longstanding, supportive friendship with Karll. Lungershausen, 19.
62. Lungershausen, 19–20. Lavinia Dock, "An Appreciation—Sister Agnes Karll," *American Journal of Nursing*, 27 (May, 1927): 357–58.
63. Lungershausen, 1964, 39.
64. Karll, 1908, 6, 51.
65. Lungershausen, 15–16; Dock, 1927, 357.
66. Karll, 1908, 6.
67. Lungershausen, 23–26.
68. Karll, 1908, 49–50.
69. Translated by Geertje Boschma: "denn von uns hatte noch nie jemand ein Protocoll aufgenommen, geschweige denn eine Versammlung geleitet." (Karll, 1908, 10).
70. Dock, 1912, 26–27.
71. Karll, 1908, 11.
72. Agnes Karll to Lavinia Dock, May 9, 1907. Letters of Karll to Dock 1907–1912. ICNA.
73. "The Great International Congress of Women at Berlin: The Nursing Section," *British Journal of Nursing*, 32 (June 25, 1904): 508–515; quotation is on 513.
74. Ibid., 513.
75. Karll, 1908, 24.
76. Letters, Agnes Karll to Lavinia Dock, 1907–1912, ICNA.
77. Kruse, 1987, 69–103.
78. The summary of the 1904 meeting in this and the following paragraphs is taken from ICN Minutes, 1899–1904, Book 1, 33–44. The quotation regarding Irish nurses is on 41.
79. Ibid., 43–44.
80. Ibid., 44.

81. L[avinia] L. Dock, "International Relationships," *Eleventh Annual Report of the American Society of Superintendents of Training Schools for Nurses . . . 1905* (Baltimore: J. H. Furst, 1905) 169–176; quotations are on 172, 173.

82. Ibid., 172–173.

83. Ibid., 173.

84. Ibid.

85. Ibid., 174.

86. Diane Hamilton, "Constructing the Mind of Nursing," *Nursing History Review*, 2, 1994: 16.

# T W O

## *The Essential Idea*

ANNE MARIE RAFFERTY
*with* Geertje Boschma

*A*s the International Council of Nurses (ICN) became more established, it sought to live up to the slogan later coined by the Northern Nurses Federation, "We are strongly individual—and together we are even stronger."[1] Promulgating a shared understanding and practice of professional nursing, and uniting nurses worldwide, however, would require a daunting and sometimes contentious attempt to unify and change a whole field of work. Caretaking of the sick was, by tradition, still firmly located in domestic and servant life, religious and missionary work, and war relief.

Nonetheless, stressing its message of unity to its constituency, the ICN, beginning in 1909, printed the following declaration as a frontispiece on all official ICN publications. Here the leaders of the ICN specified the ambitious vision of their unifying mission.

> The essential idea for which the International Council of Nurses stands, is self-government of nurses in their associations, with the aim of raising ever higher the standards of education and professional ethics, public usefulness, and civic spirit of their members. The International Council of Nurses does not stand for a narrow professionalism, but for that full development of the human being and citizen in every nurse, which shall best enable her to bring her professional knowledge and skills to the many-sided service that modern society demands of her.[2]

The ICN body politic was seen by its leaders as undivided, its voice univocal; it was a cultural commonwealth derived from a basic covenant among nurses, unfettered by national attachments, that conferred their collective power upon one assembly. Differences among nurses, although recognized, would, in this ideal scenario, be subordinated to one shared ideal.[3]

In promoting a new occupation or profession of nursing, the ICN leadership confronted a welter of beliefs about the organization of nursing work, which only partially matched their new ideals. The standards of nursing practice insisted upon by the ICN leadership often differed from the actual nursing needs within countries. ICN reformers from Western countries were influenced by changing patterns of industrial work, a new concept of occupation, and new medical techniques. Often from privileged social backgrounds, they believed in nursing as a paid professional career. As noted in the preceding chapter, most questioned nursing traditions of hierarchical authority, self-abnegation, or religious commitment. What they saw as the most advanced (Anglo-American) model of nursing was not always congruent with traditions or beliefs about care within other countries. To add to their problems, other international organizations, such as the Red Cross Societies, espoused competing practices of nursing education and work more congruent with hierarchical norms and values. This would pose a significant challenge to the proposed unifying standards of the ICN.

## Professional Prerogatives

Moreover, as they were creating their own professional agenda, the ICN leaders decided to separate themselves from the International Council of Women (ICW). Insisting on a separate ICN cannot easily be explained by the absence of a usable structure for nurses within the ICW. Fenwick was, after all, convener of the Professional Section of the ICW in 1899, and, through her, nursing was an integral part of the ICW's professional agenda.[4] Many of the cherished ideas about self-governance and regulation of standards of nursing practice were rehearsed in the pages of the ICW proceedings. Other professional groups, such as teachers, seemed content to remain within the ICW organizational framework. There is no evidence to suggest any breach or blatant division of interests between the ICN and the ICW. In fact, evidence suggests that nursing was still a subject of ICW deliberations in 1910.[5]

The relationship between the newly formed ICN and the ICW was, however, complicated by the matter of membership fees. Historian Sandra Lewenson has dissected the relationships between nursing groups in the United States, explaining the merger of the American Society of Superintendents of Training Schools for Nurses (ASSTSN) and the Nurses' Associated Alumnae of the United States and Canada to create the new American Federation of Nurses.[6] One of the reasons for their merger was to avoid double fees payable to the National Council of Women (NCW), which was the route to membership in ICW. Actually, it appears that the ICN founders saw membership in the NCW as a convenient vehicle for membership in the ICN until national nursing organizations were strong enough to organize on their own.

Some indication of this can be detected in ASSTS President Emma Keating's 1901 comment that, although the work of the NCW was interesting and instructive, it was too time-consuming for women in nursing who had so much to accomplish on their own. In 1905, the American

Federation of Nurses discontinued its 4-year membership in NCW, having joined the ICN in 1904.[7]

One could argue that the ICW had served its purpose; it had provided a valuable forum for exposing nurses to the arguments and organizational issues in suffrage and social feminism. It furnished access to networks and organizational expertise useful to the ICN. Leaving the ICW marked a turning point in the identity politics of international nursing. When membership dues "push" came to loyalty to nursing "shove," nurses had to chose between the more broadly based ICW or their special interest, the ICN. In the end, pragmatics as well as politics won the day. They decided dual membership in the ICW and ICN was a luxury organized nursing could ill afford.

## Forming the Imagined Community

The assumption that nurses' work was the same the world over underscored Fenwick's confident assertion of nursing's cultural symmetry in her 1909 address to the Second Quinquennial Meeting of the ICN. Welcoming the "glorious republic of the United States," "the great German Empire," "splendid Canada," and members from "our loyal and self-governing dominions and Colonies beyond the seas," Fenwick displayed her bias by equating civilized nations and Western countries.[8] That her view found support is evident in the article "Imperial Federation of British Nurses," cited in the New Zealand nursing journal *Kai Tiaki*. Reported to readers of Lavinia Dock's "Foreign Department" in the *American Journal of Nursing,* the authors argued that England's colonies should not have to enter the ICN as foreign states. Affiliation of all England's colonies, should, they said, all occur simultaneously at the 1909 meeting.[9] New Zealand, in particular, was perceived as a jewel in the ICN's crown, being the first country to pass a Nurse's Registration Act. Although South Africa's Cape Colony preceded New Zealand in registering nurses, doing so under the Medical and Pharmacy Act seemed a less good fit with the ICN's totemic goal of self-regulation.[10]

Equating civilization with westernization, ICN leaders reflected and reinforced contemporary views in creating their "imagined community" of nurses.[11] Indeed, ever loyal to empire, Fenwick applauded the ICN's attentions to imperial concerns. In her 1912 watchword address to the ICN's Third Regular Meeting in Cologne, Germany, she tellingly cited one of the aims of the ICN as being to "confer on questions not merely of imperial but of human weight and consequence."[12] Linking nursing's universal spiritual dimensions to the ICN's responsibility for humanity, she noted,

> The essential essence of Nursing [sic] is not merely to afford skilled help
> to suffering and diseased humanity—it is something far higher than that.

It is the endeavour to appropriate the spiritual force which is the common heritage of our profession, bequeathed to it by many noble men and women . . . so that in helping to heal the body, those to whom we minister may discern the fineness of motive which inspires our vocation, and the uplifting, spiritual zeal which inspires our service, and may be sustained and comforted thereby.[13]

Great Britain and the United States, whose organizational maturity in nursing seemed preeminent, were perceived to provide the paradigm for other organizations. "This union has been commenced in this country and the United States. It remains for the nurses of other lands to follow our example and unite amongst themselves."[14] The United States, in particular, represented itself as an example of dependence transformed into independence. In 1901, Isabel McIsaac, presiding over the Third International Congress of Nurses at the Pan-American Exposition at Buffalo, New York, had proclaimed:

To our English colleagues we of the United States owe more than we can re-pay and if in our swift American fashion we have broken from their leading strings and made paths for ourselves, we none the less acknowledge our indebtedness with gratitude, and display our accomplishments with the same pride, mingled with a little doubt with which sons and daughters display theirs to the friends at home.[15]

Ten years later, Lavinia Dock contended that the United States should provide a model of what could be achieved by less favorably placed sister countries. The purpose of international meetings, she was careful to point out, was not to have a "glorious jaunt," nor to return home "self-satisfied, complacently criticizing that which is different in other countries from our own," but to encourage nurses from other countries fighting the same battles but who "do so under a much heavier handicap than we have in our country."[16] Nationalism fused with chauvinism in Dock's proud declaration of the preeminence of the United States in international nursing affairs.

Those who fail to realize that we Americans go as a reinforcing army to strengthen the position of our allies in their campaign for a higher civilization, fail entirely to grasp the elementary meaning of the idea of "internationalism."[17]

Although the ICN leadership often seemed oblivious to their patronizing tone and the implications of their positions, their unshakeable confidence in the ideal of "empire" and the "civilizing" role of nurses as the vectors of Western bourgeois culture and values was deeply felt and shared by their constituents. Countries with colonial ties to Great Britain, such as Canada, New Zealand, and India, were among the earliest nations to join the ICN. Nor is it surprising that ICN leaders chose to locate ICN headquarters and its meetings in the cities of those colonial powers or ex-colonies, which between 1909 and 1922 occupied center stage in international politics and trade (ie, Britain, Germany and the United States).

Given the Anglo-American ideologic and practical dominance over the ICN, the influence of nursing organizations from Denmark, Finland, Germany and Holland helped it broaden its early narrow, imperialist self-concept. The ability of the northern nurses, in particular, to organize nursing associations represented the changing status of women in those countries. By 1909, for example, women in Finland had achieved suffrage; Dutch and Danish women were in the midst of independent first-wave women's movements.[18] The link between successful organization of nursing and women's organizations for social change was inextricable.

Modeling itself after the ICW, the ICN hoped to be the stimulus for nurses' national organization around the world. The ICW aimed to promote an interchange of opinion to "rouse women to new thought . . . intensify their love of liberty . . . and give them a realising sense of their power of combination."[19] Further, the ICW sought to "throw the influence of united womanhood in favour of better conditions for humanity."[20] As noted in the preceding chapter, the matching breadth of the ICN agenda was set early on by Fenwick speaking before the Council in Buffalo, New York, in 1901. The unit of organization was the graduate nurse, who would ideally gather together with her sisters through professional association for mutual help and professional progress.

> All worthy progress of women and men spring from this sense of corporate existence and reverence for political rights; associations of women to be of any real value in the body politic must comprise mind as well as matter.[21]

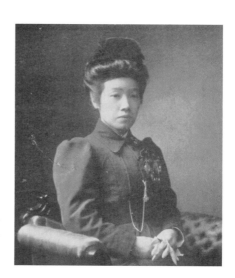

**FIGURE 2-1**
*Take Hagiwara, first Japanese Representative to the ICN, 1909. From LL Dock, History of Nursing, Vol. 4, 1912.*

During the first 20 years of this century, in addition to spreading its idea of nursing, the leadership of the ICN would focus its newly organized energy on three strands of public endeavor: the military or war effort, reforms in public health, and the ongoing suffrage movement.

## Matrons and Militarism

Officially, the ICN never advocated a pacifist position in relation to war. But, the outbreak of World War I exposed the political divisions within the ICN and split the Council between those who put their patriotic duty before their pacifist principles and those who held out for peace. Pacifism, however, was very much a minority view; one defended, almost exclusively, by Lavinia Dock, honorary secretary of the ICN, and Jeanne van Lanschot Hubrecht from Holland. Both came from countries that, initially at least, remained neutral.

Far from embracing pacifism, Fenwick and others committed to "empire," linked their arguments for equal suffrage to the premise that women could and did play an important part in warfare. In demonstrating the usefulness of the fully trained nurse to the state, Isla Stewart, president of the Matron's Council and member of the ICN Council, remarked, "To nurses alone came the honour of removing the reproach that women were of no use in time of war."[22]

From the outset, organizations pioneered by some ICN leaders sought association with the military service of the state by co-opting military nurse leaders onto their committees. This was typical of the British Nurses Association (BNA), which elected Mrs. Deeble, Lady Superintendent at Netley Naval Hospital, to the BNA executive committee in 1889.[23] Linking "professional" civilians with military nursing in the minds of officials provided a positive way of demonstrating the usefulness of nursing to the state and extracting professional recognition. Fenwick's promotion of trained and organized nursing for the state, harkened back to feminist arguments of the American Civil War and the Franco-Prussian war, according to which, women's indispensability qualified them for equal citizenship with men.[24]

As a suffragist, Fenwick insisted that war service was a powerful justification for women's political enfranchisement. Reasserting the universalist ideals of nursing she declared, "War to the death cannot affect the primary duty of the trained nurse; wherever the sick have need of us it is our duty to serve them, and we can do so the more effectively because there is no nationality in nursing."[25]

The contradictory logic of women's differential involvement yet plea for parity in the nation's work was not debated by Fenwick nor those who agreed with her. Nor was the tension between "healing" work and the human "waste" of war explored. Indeed, some argued it was the good fortune of nurses that, "while others concern themselves with matters of high policy, and may have recourse to force of arms, under no circumstances can the sick and wounded be *our* enemies."[26] There was no mention of resistance to the war or pacifism in ICN official sources; patriotism predominated. National anthems were played and sung at congresses. ICN leaders seemed to believe that far from undermining internationalism, its very existence depended on a wholesome nationalism. But, at the same time, the ICN clung to its stance that, as an international body of nurses, it should be immune to specific national concerns.

It is conceivable that the need to assert the transcendental values of internationalism was strongest at times when international relations were under pressure. Historian of British military nursing Anne Summers describes 1909 as the *annus mirabilis* of nationalist agitation, referring to the establishment of large patriotic leagues of the time, such as the Navy League and the National Service League. Although some of these formed women's sections, neither proposed that women should partake personally in national defense. However, such organizations stimulated women to establish various "vicarious" organizations of their own. The British Women's Patriotic League was one, the Women's Aerial League another.[27]

For the ICN, the key theme seemed to be that the nurses' primary loyalty was to some superordinate ideal of professionalism that went be-

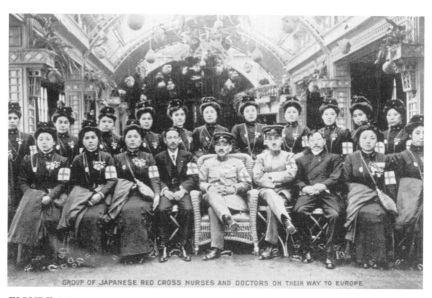

GROUP OF JAPANESE RED CROSS NURSES AND DOCTORS ON THEIR WAY TO EUROPE

*FIGURE 2-2*

*A contingent of the Japanese Red Cross enroute to Europe, 1915. From Lynaugh Collection, Bryn Mawr, PA.*

yond nationalistic concerns. In language well matched to this theme, M. Meseurer, Director of Assistance Publique in Paris, proclaimed before the ICN in Paris, 1907,

> When it is a case of nursing the sick, dressing the wounded, no one asks to what nationality they belong, but rather one admires the kind heart and hand which bring relief and comfort to suffering . . . .Frontiers do not exist for nurses. People suffer in America, in Oceania as well as in France. When a human being succumbs to illness or is lying in a hospital ward he has no country.[28]

In the United States, the national nursing organizations and the American Red Cross sought an accommodation that permitted nurses to show their national loyalty through their profession. The American Congress granted a charter in 1905 to the American Red Cross to "furnish volunteer aid to the sick and the wounded in time of war" and also to provide aid at times of natural disasters at home. Red Cross nurses would become the Army reserve in times of war, both paid and volunteer.

Affiliation of the organized nursing bodies and the Red Cross was finally worked out in 1908 when Isabel Hampton Robb proposed an administrative plan. When the United States declared war in 1917, her plan was used; 7000 nurses enrolled in the American Red Cross.[29] The American Red Cross nursing service worked primarily in France, Belgium, Italy, Romania, Palestine, and Siberia (Russia).

The work of the Department of Civil Affairs of the American Red Cross in France fell into five categories: child welfare work; establishing

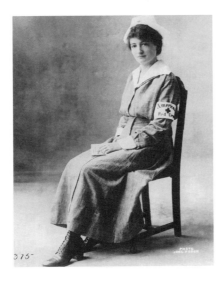

**FIGURE 2-3**
*An American Red Cross Nurse, 1916. From Lynaugh Collection, Bryn Mawr, PA.*

and maintaining homes for refugees, *rapatries,* and other exiles of war; planning for the prevention of tuberculosis throughout France; assistance to civilians returning to devastated areas; and rehabilitation of *mutiles* to help them get back to work.[30] On August 12, 1917, a pioneer American Red Cross pediatric unit, which consisted of seven physicians, one child welfare nurse and three laywomen, arrived in France to form the nucleus of personnel of the Children's Bureau. Other public health nurses already in France quickly joined the Bureau. During the war, the birth rate dropped to "forty per cent lower than the death rate," and authorities became extremely concerned about saving the remaining children and in preventing infant mortality.[31]

## Promoting the Public's Health

If most ICN leaders were ready to cooperate and participate in the war effort, they struck a more challenging note to the state when it came to public health policy. Echoing sentiments expressed in the 1907 conference in Paris, the nurse was usually conceived as *"non pas seulement un agent medical, mais un instrument de progres social et moral."*[32] By 1909, a more interventionist stance in civilian nursing was advocated within the ICN. In her opening address to the Second Quinquennial Meeting in London in 1909, Fenwick urged members of the congress to study economic conditions and take an active part in social life. She exhorted nurses to maintain a watching brief on the national health, "remembering always that a nation is only forceful so far as it is morally and physically sound."[33]

The practical implications of studying economic conditions, maintaining a watching brief on the national health, and taking an active part in social life were not acknowledged by Fenwick. Nor did she specify what exactly she meant by an active part in social life. Did she mean political campaigning on behalf of those too weak to advocate on their own behalf or did she mean only nursing reform? According to Fenwick, the nurse was more than "an instrument for the relief of suffering; she must also be the harbinger of its prevention."[34] It seemed the "war" Fenwick had in mind was to be on a broad front: "Inspired by a fine militant spirit, she will make war upon the fundamental wrongs which conduce to low vitality and physical deterioration."[35]

Fenwick's invocation of nurses' so-called militant spirit was also ambiguous. Was she referring to the activism of the suffragists led by the Pankhursts or merely seeking a tactical turn of phrase for the benefit of R. B. Haldane, Secretary of State for War, who addressed the same meeting on the connection between war nursing and women's emancipation? This ambiguity may well have been deliberate because suffragists were active in London at the time of the meeting. Dock had publicized cases of suffragist nurses, imprisoned for their part in campaigns the previous year.[36]

She reported instances of nurses who had been subjected to force-feeding, a practice deplored by Sir Victor Horsley, distinguished surgeon and ally of Fenwick, as potentially gravely injurious to health. Horsley led a protest containing the signatures of other prominent physicians and addressed to the Prime Minister. Nurses raised objections to what they regarded as the "degradation of the healing art and of one of its last resorts for the preservation of life, in being used to as a brutal method to suppress free speech and the demands for justice."[37] Dock proclaimed, "Some day the whole nursing profession will be as proud of these patriots as the world now is of Jeanne, D'Arc who has recently been sainted."[38] Using religious rhetoric, she extolled the virtues of the "martyrs serving prison sentences and hard labor in the cause of setting women free . . . ."[39]

Throughout Secretary Haldane's speech to the ICN Congress, he was hectored by assembled suffragists, who, there solely to demand votes, were uninterested in his views on the likelihood of war, or the implications of his schemes, such as the Territorial Army Service, for the future role of women in society.[40] Interestingly, this important, and possibly embarrassing, episode was not included in either the ICN reports of the meeting or the history subsequently produced by Fenwick and Margaret Breay.

Fenwick's 1909 speech also touched on the prevailing mood of anxiety surrounding Britain's future as an imperial power. She urged sensitivity on the part of the fully trained nurse to the needs of the state. For instance, the British government's Physical Deterioration Committee had, 4 years earlier, revealed the prevalence of "degenerative" disease among army recruits to the Boer War. Social diseases and moral lassitude were identified as the key contributors to the vitiation of Britain's "racial stock." The official response to the findings of the Physical Deterioration Committee was to improve health supervision and surveillance of working class districts in urban areas. Sanitary and later health visiting and public health nursing emerged as key collaborators in trying to eradicate the dual evils of poverty and disease.

The Second Quinquennial Conference included a number of papers calling for a broadly based social and political agenda for nursing and the civic engagement of nurses.[41] In addition to Secretary Haldane's speech on The Nurse as Patriot, and The Nurse as Citizen by Lady Munro Ferguson, contributions included The Nurse among the Poor by Mlle. Leonie Chaptal; Nursing in Prisons, by Fenwick; and Social Service in Connection With Hospitals, by Annie Goodrich.[42]

In her paper, Lady Munro Ferguson called for a liberal definition of nursing work locating it within a framework of national importance. She proclaimed that, "even in nursing's most menial task lay work of humanitarian and civic importance."

When she ministers to the poorest old chronic, let her see herself representing that common brotherhood which binds society together:

when she struggles for the eyesight of one poor fretful baby, let her see herself fighting for national efficiency.[43]

It was within this context that Fenwick identified the public health nurse as a solution to the state's twin problems of moral malaise and malady. Decrying the parochialism of hospital training she remarked,

> The practice of nursing in the future will not be restricted to a few years' mechanical training in hospital wards, and subsequently to a more or less narrow sphere of influence, but under a comprehensive curriculum defined by State authority, it will attain a definite value to the community. So much of the moral welfare of the people depends upon sanitary conditions that a nurse who grasps her opportunities could find herself in touch with her relief of human suffering.[44]

Public health nursing was thus promoted by Fenwick as an alternative model of citizenship to that of military nursing. Just as the character of the community in which the new nurse would serve was in the throes of reconstruction, so too was the identity of the nurse. The ideal nurse of the future would be beyond reproach in terms of her moral and social qualifications, her sense of civic duty and responsibility. As Fenwick proclaimed,

> Only those can hope to excel in our profession who possess refined and cultured breeding, a liberal education, vigorous physical energy, noble qualities of the mind, deep well-springs of human sympathy, gracious manners, a sensitive public spirit, and a splendid conviction of right.[45]

Public health provided a powerful metaphor and mechanism by which the ICN could forge a rapprochement between the aims of the state and organized nursing. During the 1909 Congress, a notable number of papers reflected contemporary public health concerns under the rubric of "Morality in Relation to Health." In an impassioned plea to the congress to fight against the "paralysing indifference" to the ravages of venereal disease, the Honorable Albinia Broderick from the National Council of Nurses of Great Britain inveighed against the hypocrisy and neglect surrounding its prevention.[46] Education for children in sexual physiology and inculcation of self-discipline were identified as key resources in the fight against venereal disease. Removal of the moral stigma attached to treatment and reduction of alcoholism were also considered important interventions. Such so-called progressive measures were combined with recommendations to punish any infected person who knowingly exposed another to risk of infection.[47] Enumerating enemies of public health as "the ignorant, the prudish, the timid, the vicious, the alcoholic, the feeble-minded (and) . . . mock modesty of any kind," Broderick called for nurses to act on their behalf using "knowledge, unity and love" as weapons for attack and victory.[48] Dock endorsed the importance and urgency of the crusade and deplored the venereal scourge as the consequence of the "servile acceptance of a double standard of morals, one for men and one for women."[49]

Education was deemed the essential weapon against overcoming prudery and thereby the spread of disease. Reducing prostitution and the white slave trade were assigned first priority.[50] The message was carried through to the resolution stage of the congress, each national organization being exhorted to appoint in its own country a standing committee on morality and public health to explore a number of areas over which nurses could exercise some influence and jurisdiction. These areas of influence included: the extent to which immorality was affected by national or local laws, recommending suitable instruction material on the matter, communicating with national societies on moral prophylaxis, and petitioning for hospital nurses to receive teaching on such matters.[51] The relationship between social hygiene and health became the subject of a book published by Dock and the substance of a proposal from her that each country should appoint a standing committee on morality and health to formulate national strategies for action.[52]

The ICN successfully identified itself with and courted the support and approval of the military and public health authorities. And, by 1912, this new rhetoric of responsiveness to community needs was being propagated by the ICN to justify the reform of nursing education.

In April 1919, after the Armistice, the Cannes conference met to decide on and prioritize the work to be undertaken by the national Red Cross societies. Out of this conference grew the League of Red Cross Societies (LRCS). The members stressed the necessity for nurses to be competent in public health nursing. However, according to American Clara Noyes, "the emphasis was placed on the establishment of schools of nursing." Subsequently, the Red Cross, especially the American Red Cross, started and maintained schools of nursing in many eastern European countries devastated both by war and their preexisting poverty, such as Romania, Yugoslavia, Poland, and Bulgaria. Each of these schools had American or British directors. Standards varied tremendously partly because, in many countries, nursing was seen as a menial service fit for only the lower classes.

As Noyes observed in Prague in 1920, facilities for teaching were often grossly inadequate, as were food allowances for students and even bars of soap, which were strictly rationed to two bars per ward for all cleaning and washing purposes.[53] Nevertheless, this postwar investment in nursing would importantly affect the later size and scope of the ICN. At local and national levels, ICN leaders sought opportunities to visit state-controlled centers of health care. Such visits and congresses helped to forge unions with strategically important allies and authorities.

## Suffrage and Citizenship

The third strand of public endeavor that the ICN employed in its strategy was suffrage. Even if nursing was supposed to be a nationally neutral phenomenon, it was nevertheless class- and gender-specific. Fenwick argued, "We need the very flower of womanhood to maintain these ideals."[54] Registration for trained nurses and suffrage for all women were inextricably mixed in the minds of ICN leaders and the subject of two consecutive resolutions in 1909.[55] The ICN's commitment to registration and women's suffrage was reiterated at the Third Business Meeting in Cologne in 1912.

Yet, unlike the international labor movement, there was no threat from the ICN to impose sanctions against governments who failed to provide for registration. Arguments were essentially moral, implying governments' duty to care by protecting the public from fraudulent and incompetent nurses; and, of course, by protecting trained nurses from the untrained. With respect to the question of suffrage, the 1912 resolution read,

> We . . . regard the suffrage movement as a great moral movement making for the conquest of misery, preventable illness, and vice, and as strengthening a feeling of human brotherhood.[56]

Here can be seen collapsing of categories so that any boundaries between the moral mission of womanhood, suffrage, public health nursing and social hygiene were broken down and merged into a unifying ideology.

The 1909 Parliamentary Franchise suffrage resolution proposed by the Netherlands' Hubrecht, an ardent supporter of women's suffrage, offered its "sincere and respectful congratulations to the women, and especially to the trained nurses, in those Countries and States in which they have been granted the rights of citizenship."[57] It was seconded by Finland's Baroness Mannerheim. Both the Baroness and Susan McGahey, from Australia, preempted and countered criticisms that women would not use the vote if granted.[58] MacLean from New Zealand was more cautious. Although women had had the vote since 1893, she claimed no nurses took an active part in politics. Perhaps, she thought, it was because their work was too absorbing and those engaged in private nursing found it difficult to extricate themselves from their duties with private patients.[59] These comments foreshadowed the future disappointments of suffrage workers who found that, even with the vote, women failed to make a political impact.[60]

That the initiative for the Parliamentary Franchise resolution arose from an individual and not from a national association where the franchise had already been granted or, indeed, from a suffragist member of the Grand Council may seem strange. On the other hand, for the issue to be raised by a member from a country where suffrage did not exist might well cast doubt on the legitimacy of her leadership on the matter. So, for the resolution to come from outside the Council, does not mean that ICN executive leaders were either against or unsympathetic to suffrage—far from it.

Ethel Gordon Fenwick was a well-known suffragist, being a subscriber to the militant Women's Social and Political Union (WSPU). Headed by Mrs. Pankhurst in 1903, the WSPU worked to promote women's interests within the labor movement from 1908 to 1914.[61] Fenwick's *British Journal of Nursing* had petitioned for Nurse Pitfield to be released from prison after a militant demonstration in London and allegedly led a fund-raising campaign to achieve this.[62] Similarly, Dock, on one of her many trips to England, volunteered her services to Pankhurst in February 1914.[63] Dock urged readers of her *American Journal of Nursing* Foreign Department column to heed the resolutions passed by the first Quinquennial Conference of the International Woman Suffrage Alliance and quoted these in full, providing a review of the position of suffrage in each of the 21 member countries.[64]

Links between registration and suffrage continued to resonate through ICN deliberations, including at the Third Triennial Meeting in Cologne in 1912, where a resolution was passed conflating the objectives of suffrage with social hygiene and national efficiency movements. The overlapping functions and blurred boundaries between social work and nursing were noted in a number of papers at the Cologne meeting. These included discussion of the social service of the nurse, the care of orphans, the work of the police assistant, homes for working women and welfare work for consumptive patients, health visitors and sanitary inspectors.[65] The suffrage movement, fusing the humanitarian goals of public health, was memorialized by ICN leaders as a "great moral movement making for the conquest of misery, preventable illness and vice, and as strengthening a feeling of human brotherhood."[66]

## Obstacles to Implementing the ICN Idea

Although the ICN Council consistently agreed on its own essential idea of nursing, it found itself handicapped in two ways: not only did delegates have to deal with different languages but, if the council were to fulfill one of its chief aims, "to confer upon questions relating to the welfare of their patients," some consensus had to be reached on how to conceptualize nursing problems.[67] One way to realize their unifying ideology, they believed, was through the invention of an international language of nursing. The proposal for a "Nursing Esperanto" first appeared in the paper by Mrs. Hampton Robb on the International Education Standard for Nurses delivered in London at the Second Quinquennial Meeting in 1909. Hampton Robb thought a common language of nursing would be necessary to universalize nurse training methods and facilitate their communication throughout the nursing world.[68] Close to 80 years would pass before any action was taken on her proposal.

Another troubling problem was the variation in the chronology and content of nurses' training revealed in a survey of preliminary training schools conducted by Dock and Sister Agnes Karll and various reports on state registration and developments in training in Great Britain, the United States, New Zealand, Germany, Belgium, Italy and Hungary.[69] For example, in the United States, it was alleged there were not more than five institutions prepared to give the recommended standard of 6 months' preliminary course under qualified instruction.[70] So great was the gap between the better and worse general hospitals under private management in the United States, it was claimed "pages" would be needed to describe it.[71]

ICN speakers decried lack of standards across and within national nurse associations as impediments to the development of collegial relationships. Anger and frustration at the exploitative policies and attitudes of hospital management committees toward probationers, both as a cheap form of labor and source of income, led Karll, among others, to establish professional organizations in the first place. What was required, but lacking, was system and regularity in teaching nursing, in which theoretical and practical instruction throughout the duration of training could be combined.[72] This high degree of variation from the stated standards, more than anything else, underlines that the ICN was more a congeries of different parts moving at different speeds than a composite whole.

Attaining mobility for nurses in an unregulated labor market was an important premise underpinning the drive for nurse registration. Uniform standards of education and registration were assumed to be prerequisites to international mobility and migration of nurses. ICN leaders believed that, if nursing was to become internationalized, first it had to be standardized.

## Taking a Position on Working Conditions

Prominent among Karll's priorities as the incoming ICN president was curbing the occupational mortality and morbidity of nurses. Part of her interest may well have stemmed from her own ill health in 1901 after several arduous years as a private-duty nurse in Berlin.[73] The problem of high levels of morbidity and mortality in nurses was particularly acute after the expansion of insurance-based welfare programs in Europe increased the demand for nurses, which training schools were struggling to meet.

Although religious sisterhoods were considered particularly vulnerable to exploitation and overpressure of work, concern was expressed for all types of nurses, because most were excluded from insurance coverage.[74]

In fact, in England, insurance in case of unemployment applied only to a small number of trades, from which women were mainly excluded.[75] For the purposes of insurance, nurses were classed as domestic and not professional workers. Along with all other women who might be insured, they apparently paid a higher rate for benefits than men.[76]

Given this situation and the interests of the ICN leadership, it is no coincidence that the subject of one of the first ICN position papers was the effects of physical strain and fatigue on nurses' health.[77] Such research was consistent with a more general concern expressed through the welfarist humanitarian researches of such employers as Cadbury and Rowntree.[78] In the United States, the efficiency movement, born out of the enthusiasm for scientific management, fueled reaction already generated by the findings of the *Report of the Inter-departmental Committee on Physical Deterioration, 1904–5* in Britain. Within Britain, it was the health of women workers, particularly those working within the munitions industry, that finally provoked the establishment of the Industrial Fatigue Research Board in 1918 and the development of physiologic measurement in industrial psychology research.[79] In her column, Dock also applauded the pioneering work undertaken by the Italians in the scientific study of fatigue and pernicious effects of overwork on health in general.[80]

Although nursing was not considered an archetypically dangerous trade, it is significant that it was one of the first female-dominated occupations with claims to professionalism to be the subject of contemporary research in industrial psychology. There was a sense, therefore, in which the ICN was courting controversy and undermining its own claims to professionalism by identifying with a form of research more usually associated with the industrial or trade sector. But ICN leaders were caught on the horns of a dilemma because industrial psychology promised to provide a powerful means of generating scientifically respectable evidence with which to fight for reforms. This was particularly relevant to the practice of private-duty nursing, which was notoriously prone to exploitation due to the domesticated or hidden nature of the nurse–patient (working) relationship. Private nurses were an important constituency in registrationists' armamentarium and arguments. Determining the exact nature of their work, therefore, not only served to protect nurses from unfair disadvantage but helped define the work of nursing as distinct from that of other disciplines.

## The Matter of Miss Nightingale

It was also at the Cologne conference that Fenwick announced the desire of some delegates to establish a memorial to Miss Nightingale in the form of an educational bequest. Nightingale was characterized as being above nationality, belonging to every age and country, and endowed with the genius to realize that nursing must follow scientific medicine as its hand-maid. Fenwick appeared to overlook any contradiction such a proposition might pose for emancipatory ideals of professionalism because Nightingale was neither in favor of registration nor suffrage for women, believing property rights should take precedence over the franchise in determining women's independence. However, it is often in the nature of the post hoc reconstruction of heroism that characteristics are attributed to individuals that they do not possess and might reject.[81] Such was Nightingale's iconic status that a banner with the word "Crimea" headed the 500-strong nursing contingent of a suffragist parade in London, dressed in uniform and led by Fenwick.[82]

## The War Years

After the Cologne meeting and following an invitation from the California Nurses' Association, it was decided to hold the next conference in San Francisco in conjunction with the American Nurses' Association Convention and the 1915 Panama-Pacific Exposition.[83] The decision to hold the next meeting in San Francisco followed the election of Annie Goodrich, Inspector of Training Schools in New York, as ICN president for the next triennial term. The opportunity to be part of the Panama-Pacific Exposition was seen by the ICN as a public endorsement of nursing as being among the leading associations of thinkers and workers in the world.[84]

Dock was, of course, heavily involved in planning the details of the 1915 Congress. Adelaide Nutting and Annie Goodrich traveled to Eng-

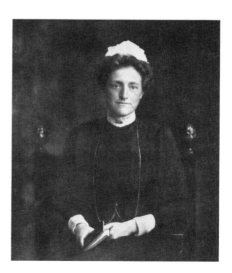

*FIGURE 2-4*
*Annie Goodrich, ICN President 1912 to 1915. From AJN Collection.*

land during August 1914, stopping in London to discuss ICN business on their way to a tour of the Continent. By August 15, however, their trip cut short by the outbreak of war, they returned to the United States, Nutting on a freight ship from Glasgow to New York by way of Newfoundland.[85]

No records of the wartime activities of the ICN remain, except what was published in relevant journals and sources such as Bridges' history. Many of the national nursing ICN leaders from Europe and her colonies became involved in relief work during the war. Their involvement in any other activities ground to a standstill. As Dock lamented in 1915,

> The darkness of this terrible war is repeated in the silence of our European members. Not a line has come from any country in Europe since the war broke out, except a brief note from Miss Hubrecht in Holland . . . . She fears not more than two or three can hope to attend the San Franciscan Congress instead of the dozen or more who planned to do so from Holland.[86]

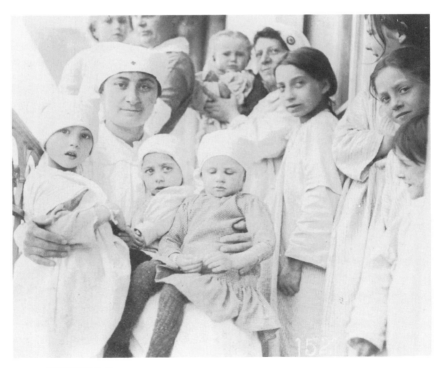

**FIGURE 2-5**
*Red Cross nurses with World War 1 child refugees (Lynaugh Collection, Bryn Mawr, PA).*

In view of the continuing demands of war, suffrage campaigning, and the incongruity of celebrating any form of international day at the congress, the wisdom of holding a regular meeting of the ICN in San Francisco in 1915 was questioned.[87] Work continued on ICN business by the American Committee of the ICN. However, they suspended work on raising funds to support a chair in nursing, which they hoped would form the basis of the memorial to Nightingale.[88] Instead, they focused on planning the next full meeting of the ICN in the neutral territory of Copenhagen in 1918.

Even at the height of World War I, ICN leaders confidently clung to their commitment that nursing was neutral in matters of national interest. Readers of the *British Journal of Nursing* were reminded that "no shadow of bitterness toward one another can possibly arise. The sick and wounded, friend or enemy, is our sacred charge and any woman who can harbour an unkind feeling for any soldier who falls at his country's call, little appreciates either a soldiers' duty or her own." This sentiment was of particular consequence to German nurses, who were viewed as victims rather than accomplices in Germany's war effort.

> For our part we have thought much and in deep sympathy with dear Sister Agnes Karll, and our many German sisters, whose kindness and generosity to us . . . that were we to meet them all again, in a neutral world across the Atlantic, it would indeed be a cause for rejoicing. If Peace has come by June 1915, the members of the German Nurses Association will, we know, be as happy to greet us in international amity at San Francisco as the delegates of the great British Confederation of Nurses from home and overseas will be to greet them.[89]

Implicit within these declarations is the sense that women and, therefore, nurses should be exonerated from any responsibility for the evils of war, because they had no part in its political determination.

On the other hand, the war emergency kindled the tendency among the professionalizing contingent within the ICN to vent their spleen against what Dock and others saw as the "snobbish, amateur, and untrained Red Cross society lady nurses."[90] Dock denounced harshly the Red Cross Societies of some foreign countries as women engaged "in the great game of glory-hunting, [just] as war gives men of their class the most exciting game on earth."[91] Dock was especially critical of any nurse's tendency to be drawn into what she referred to as a 'theatrical pageant,' glorifying war and identifying with militarism and militaristic ideals.[92]

In attacking the Red Cross, Dock was, to some extent, attacking her own kind. Fenwick, for example, worked with the British Red Cross, trying to reform from within, fighting for higher standards of training. It is clear that among ICN leaders, Dock's was a minority point of view. Most of her European sisters were engaged in Red Cross or other war-related work.

An exception was Hubrecht, who shared Dock's pacifist position. Holland, along with Denmark, remained neutral in the war. Hubrecht believed nurses should take up a much more critical and adversarial position in relation to war. She condemned the complicitous role of nursing's involvement in war and advocated instead that nurses should strike against war or nurse only those soldiers who, upon regaining their health, would go back to work and not to the front.[93]

Both Hubrecht and Dock blamed the war on men's greed and competitive impulses. They called into question men's right to govern given the horrendous consequences that such characteristics engendered. They edged toward recommending that women not only disengage from the institutions associated with war, but turn their backs on the failed system of secret diplomacy, working toward a new diplomacy and world order, founded not on competition (shorthand for the capitalist system) but cooperation.[94] Regrettably, Hubrecht would not live to strive further for peace; she died shortly after the war's end in 1919.[95]

Meanwhile only a few delegates made their way to San Francisco to attend the business meeting of the ICN. It was hoped that the meeting could maintain some kind of solidarity and continuity in the ICN's affairs throughout the troubled period of the war. Dock saw the purpose of the meeting as being

> to save our international union from the stupid mania of destruction, suspicion and hatred that is now sweeping the earth under the false titles of "patriot," "honor," "defense of country," and all other specious phrases used by men to deck their deeds of piracy, land-grabbing, highway robbery and murder.[96]

Yet she would not be present at the meeting, devoting herself instead to the efforts of the suffrage movement, which she considered the necessary

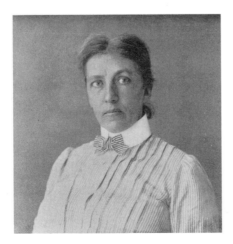

**FIGURE 2-6**
*Jeanne van Lanschot Hubrecht, President of the Dutch Nurses Association. From LL Dock, History of Nursing, Vol. 4, 1912.*

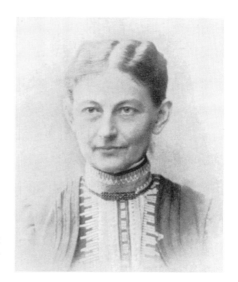

**FIGURE 2-7**
*Henny Tscherning, ICN President 1915 to 1922. From LL Dock, History of Nursing, Vol. 3, 1912.*

precondition of registration.[97] Not one to miss an opportunity to ventilate her views, Dock ensured that a speaker from the Congressional Union for Woman Suffrage would address the 600 participants in the convention.[98]

In her presidential address, Goodrich was careful not to make value judgments about the war except to refer to it as a "terrible tragedy."[99] Election of Danish Council of Nurses' President Mrs. Henny Tscherning to be ICN president more clearly articulated their eagerness for peace and neutrality.

Shortly after becoming a nurse in 1878, Tscherning was appointed as a wardwoman and later head nurse at a new surgical ward of one of the Copenhagen hospitals. She worked closely with the medical staff to introduce new antiseptic treatments on the ward. During this time, she spent some weeks at St. Thomas Hospital in London to study the new methods of nursing. After her marriage, she stopped practicing and continued her nursing activities as a leader of the Danish Council of Nurses, in which she remained active for the next 25 years.[100] The Danish Council of Nurses influenced and, in turn, was influenced by both its British and German "sisters."

Passage of the mantle of leadership to Mrs. Tscherning was further accented by the fact that, for the first time, Fenwick, Breay and Karll as well as Dock were absent from an ICN gathering.

## Lurking Shades

It is clear from some of the early mission statements that ICN leaders saw the organization as being invested with some kind of quasilegal status. Fenwick argued that the ICN should become the "deliberative assembly and supreme court of appeal of the nursing world."[101] This does seem to presuppose disputes were likely to occur or would require mediation or arbitration. Dock, writing in 1919, gives us some insight into the prevailing tensions between member countries, which arose from national political differences.

> From the beginning of the time when nurses met in international relations, there have always been present under the surface at these meetings, lurking shades cast by the political outlines of their nationalities. While these were so well concealed as to be only perceived by sensitive natures, still they were there.[102]

As will be seen in Chapter 3, Irish, Finnish, Korean, and Chinese nurses all had justifiable grudges against the policies and imperialistic incursions of certain sister ICN countries.

Here also Dock made the first public allusion to racial and ethnic issues within countries as a potential source of contention and division in the ICN. Referring to the 1907 Paris meeting, Dock drew attention to the paradox of "negro" nurses from the United States, who attended the meeting and there enjoyed a level of personal respect and absence of prejudice denied to them in their own country.[103] Like black nurses in South Africa, African Americans were barred from membership in their national associations.[104]

Earlier, the *American Journal of Nursing* singled out the 1912 Congress in Cologne for comment as an example of the assimilationist ethos of the ICN, because the affiliation of the National Association of Nurses of India marked not only a meeting of East with West, but the inclusion of an association that offered membership to so-called native nurses.[105] At the same meeting, however, Karll's impulsive toast to peace provoked only a half-hearted response—while the French absented themselves entirely from the Cologne sessions.[106]

Try as they might to smooth over political differences among nations, the ICN was striving against a time of great social upheaval. Nowhere does the real meaning of this become more obvious than in the case of Russia.

## The Russian Example

Russia never became a member of the ICN, although some scattered international contacts developed early in the 20th century.[107] The Russian example is a reminder that one of the most important factors determining whether a country could link with the ICN was the presence of international nursing contacts that fit Anglo-American ideals. One of the basic tenets of the ICN was the formation of a national independent nursing organization, characterized by self-organization and able to link with the ICN. Such an organization never developed in Russia.

The most influential organization of Russian nurses until World War I and the revolutionary changes of 1917 was the Russian Red Cross Society. During the Crimean War, groups of women organized themselves to care for wounded soldiers on the battlefields. One of their leaders, Elizabeth Kartzeff, founded a school of nursing in St. Petersburg in 1854, after the war was over. This school, soon followed by many others, adopted the nursing model of the time; that is, nurses trained and practiced under church protection and doctrine. On entry to the 2-year training program, the student understood she would become a Sister of Mercy, bind herself to the school's sisterhood, and give up her personal life. The school (or motherhouse, comparable to the German model) was responsible for her material and moral life; matrons supervised the nurses as a mother would her family.

After the founding of the Russian Red Cross in the late 19th century, many of these schools came under its patronage, and formal training and examination were introduced, although the graduates kept the title of Sister of Mercy and religious life remained a prominent part of the organization.[108] By 1914, there were 109 Red Cross schools in Russia.[109]

During the 20th century, Russia began to develop another system of training for more educated nurses called *felschers* (or *fledshers*) for male nurses and *felscheritza* (female nurses). These nurses were trained to assist physicians in 2- or 3-year programs in large hospitals. The students paid for their education and were paid salaries as soon as they obtained a position.[110] Even though these fledshers seemingly shared characteristics that were part of the standard ICN image of nurses, Lavinia Dock, ICN secretary, sounded negative as she discussed the Red Cross nurses and the fledshers in her 1909 report on Russian nursing in the *American Journal of Nursing*. She argued that they "have not as dignified nor authoritative positions as our [American] head nurses, nor quite the same responsibility."[111] Neither the Red Cross nursing model nor the fledsher model matched the ICN ideal.

The radical changes of the 1917 October revolution deeply affected medical service in Russia. The Bolshevik government reformed health care according to Communist policy. As with all other workers, health personnel were required to join a large union.[112] Unlike their western European counterparts, Communist unions were not self-governing nor could they bargain for better working conditions or use strikes. Unions for health personnel had to contribute to industrial production and improve health administration.[113] The political transition destroyed existing organizations such as the Russian Red Cross and other established educational institutions.[114] As of 1921, new schools of nursing were founded with totally different professional standards and with curriculums according to the Communist model.[115]

## Coping With Political Realities

The Russian example highlights the formidable obstacles confronting the worldwide organizational aspirations of the ICN. The ICN leadership also seemed to fear that the ICN could become "infected" with the sectarian politics that beset the pursuit of nursing reform in national contexts.[116] Unity of purpose, although always sought in national associations, was no foregone conclusion. Dock had a longstanding anxiety, for example, that the ICN would fall prey to the fissiparous politics of nursing organizations in England. As early as 1901, after the Congress at Buffalo, she lamented the "diverse cliques in England . . . (who) keep the 'Ego' too much to the front."[117] However, she qualified her statement by adding that any apparent divisions were mostly based on personal preferences, not on ultimate purposes.

Although there were plans to hold a full meeting of the ICN in Copenhagen in 1918, communications were disrupted, and the social, political, and economic shocks of the war took their toll. Dock complained that the only way she could receive letters from Tscherning, president of the ICN, was by way of a Danish nurse passing through New York. These included copies of letters written over a year ago but never received.[118] Instead, an effort was made to gather the ICN executives in 1920 at Atlanta, Georgia at the convention of the American Nurses Association. But only a small number of delegates from the ICN went to Atlanta; the delegates from Britain were busy contending with recently passed legislation on nurses' registration.

Although Tscherning was forced to serve as ICN president under trying wartime conditions, she nonetheless continued to promote nursing in the northern European countries. For example, Tscherning was one of the initiators of the idea of international exchange between the northern

INFLUENZA

Beginning in 1918, an influenza pandemic swept through North America and Europe, spread from the United States to Europe by the migration of armies. It particularly seemed to devastate young adults. As the war drew to a close, it swept across Germany, paralyzing domestic life and the war effort. In three terrible waves—July 1918, October 1918, and February 1919—millions of North Americans and Europeans died. Estimates suggest more than 40 million people in the world died; this toll was higher than any previous recorded pandemic in history.

European countries and helped establish the Northern Nurses Federation (NNF), which first met in 1920 in Copenhagen.[119] Three nurses from each of the four national associations in the NNF, Denmark, Finland, Norway, and Sweden, met every 3 years to discuss important issues relevant to the nursing profession, such as the 3-year training program, the economic conditions of nurses and the 8-hour work day, nursing ethics, and nursing and social work and child welfare. Iceland would later join the NNF in 1923.[120]

The ICN meeting scheduled for Copenhagen finally took place in 1922 but involved only the Grand Council. Among the countries represented at Copenhagen were Denmark, Great Britain and Ireland, the United States, Finland, Holland, India, Belgium, Italy, Norway, South Africa, and Iceland. The absence of Germany and Canada was regretted, due to factors of distance in the case of Canada, and the low exchange rate in the case of Germany.

Fenwick sent her apologies and welcomed new countries seeking affiliation; Belgium, China, Italy, Norway, and South Africa joined the great fellowship of nurses.[121] Among the factors that made this an enjoyable conference was relief at escaping from the strain of war-torn countries into neutral territory, which had not experienced the extreme deprivations of war. One commentator especially enthused about the food, noting its plentiful supply and delicious tastes.[122] The 1922 meeting was a landmark because it also marked the passing of the old guard. Dock resigned after 22 years as honorary secretary of the ICN. Baroness Sophie Mannerheim of Finland was elected as president for the next session.[123]

One of the primary issues on the agenda of the meeting was the question of mobility and migration of nurses between countries. Maude MacCallum, long-time ally of Fenwick and representative from Great Britain, proposed that each affiliated country be asked to collect information on which hospitals in that country would be prepared to receive foreign probationers.[124] This issue was also under consideration by the Ministry of Health in Great Britain.[125]

It seems that the ICN was considering developing a role as a kind of international labor exchange aiming at the "internationalisation" of nursing labor. As a trade union leader, MacCallum was likely to be sensitive to such issues. A further concern may have been the desire to use nurse registration as a means of rationalizing nursing qualifications, using probationer labor in exchange programs as a lever in the struggle to standardize approaches to nursing education and practice.[126] Indeed, a resolution was passed recommending that information on courses available to foreign probationers should be collated by the international secretary.[127] How such a task might be accomplished given the lack of staff and resources of the ICN was left unresolved.

A further issue connected with nursing labor related to the question of the length of the work week.[128] This debate was part of a more general debate raging within the trade union movement in Great Britain and raised more fundamental questions concerning the status of nursing either as a self-regulating profession or regulated industrial work.[129] Opinion and practice varied on the matter. Some advocated a weekly limit of 54 hours per week, fearing nurses would lose the esteem and support of the public if they reduced their daily hours. A standard reduction to a 54-hour week was adopted as a council resolution, but many favored the 8-hour day, particularly to protect the interests of probationers and others prone to overwork, poor health, and exploitation.[130] A similar debate had dragged on in the United States for at least 40 years. Likewise, nurses in the NNF struggled with the 8-hour day as compromising nursing's ethical base and ideology. There was general agreement to shorten the work week but limited support for the 8-hour day.[131]

The cognate issue of setting an international standard for nursing education was resuscitated in a paper given by Miss Pearse from Great Britain. Isabel Hampton Robb had introduced the subject in 1909 but died unexpectedly in 1910. The Secretary of the Committee on Nursing Education, Hubrecht, died in 1919, leaving Adelaide Nutting as the only remaining member of the original standing committee.

Guidance was sought from the council on the duration of training; the standard curriculum drawn up by the Committee on Nursing Education chaired by Nutting was commended. The need to define the criteria of quality in educational programs seemed especially important because nursing was under increasing pressure to compete with other occupational options for female recruits. Pearse, in her opening address to the Fourth Regular Meeting of the ICN remarked,

> Education . . . is the rock on which we are in danger of foundering. At present the failure of nursing to attract women of education and intelligence is a very real difficulty. How can it be remedied? By showing intelligent and educated girls that nursing is a satisfying and remunerative career.[132]

Standardization of education became not only a matter for the probationer, but now extended to specialist postgraduate courses in public health and welfare, mental nursing, midwifery and district nursing.[133] Collaboration with women's colleges was encouraged. Courses offered in public health nursing at Bedford College for Women and the London County Council School Nursing Service (with which Pearse was associated) were held up as models for emulation. These were suggested as a possible focus for international exchange programs. This latter idea was an initiative that would finally come to fruition in the mid 1930s under the auspices of the Florence Nightingale International Foundation (FNIF).[134]

# After Two Decades

Dogged by problems of limited resources and unstable international politics and relations, the ICN was frustrated in its efforts to realize its "imagined community" ideals.[135] Yet its leadership was, at the same time, alert to the discrepancy that might arise between aspiration and achievement. In her watchword address to the Third Regular Meeting in Cologne, Fenwick had admitted, "From its inception our Council has aspired far beyond what was considered practicable."[136]

The challenges confronting the ICN were, indeed, formidable as nursing became embroiled in wider international politics and conflict. Lacking any solid legal or diplomatic status, the ICN, nevertheless, provided a vital frame of reference and leverage that nurses around the world could use for professional regulation and to press for precious resources and reform. The extent to which the ICN succeeded in transcending its avowed fear of narrow professionalism, "raising even higher the standards of . . . public usefulness and civic spirit of their members" and reaching for their "essential idea" needs to be measured in this light.[137]

## ENDNOTES

1. Nete Balslev Wingender, "We Are Strongly Individual and Together We Are Even Stronger," *International History of Nursing Journal*, 1(4): 77–87. The Northern Nurses Federation consists of the professional nurses' associations of Denmark, Finland, Norway, Sweden, and Iceland; it was founded in 1920 to ensure good quality nursing education and fair working conditions for nurses.

2. Frontispiece, Second Quinquennial Meeting of the International Council of Nurses, London, 1909. ICNA.

3. See Kathleen B. Jones, *Compassionate Authority: Democracy and the Representation of Women* (New York: Routledge, 1993) for a fuller discussion of how the transcendence of difference in democracies leads to authority.

4. International Congress of Women, *Women in Professions*, 1900.

5. *Report of the International Congress of Women Held in Toronto, Canada 1909* (Parker: Toronto, 1910).

6. Sandra Lewenson, "'Of Logical Necessity . . . They Hang Together,' Nursing and the Women's Movement, 1901–1912," *Nursing History Review*, 2 (1994): 99–118.

7. For a review of the complex choreography of organizational arrangements and alignments, see Sandra Lewenson, *Taking Charge: Nursing, Suffrage, and Feminism in America, 1873–1920* (New York: Garland Press, 1993), 91–101.

8. Second Quinquennial Meeting, 1909. ICNA.

9. Lavinia Dock, "Foreign Department: International Congress,"*American Journal of Nursing*, 9 (September 1909): 674.

10. "The New Zealand Trained Nurses Association," *British Journal of Nursing* (August 3, 1912): 88.

11. Anderson, *Imagined Communities*, 6. The use of "imagined community" is Anderson's way of defining the image that fellow members of nations have of each other in spite of the fact that they may never meet or really know each other.

12. Third Regular Meeting of the International Council of Nurses, Cologne, 1912, The Triennial Meeting, 14. ICNA.

13. Third Business Meeting of the International Council of Nurses, Cologne, 1912, The Triennial Meeting, 14. ICNA.

14. ICN Records Book 2, 1899–1904, excerpt from *British Journal of Nursing,* 1899, n.d., ICNA.

15. Breay and Fenwick, 21. Miss McIsaac opening the 1901 Congress at Buffalo.

16. Lavinia Dock, "Foreign Department: Plans for the Cologne Congress," *American Journal of Nursing,* 11 (November 1911): 9, 719–720.

17. Ibid., 20.

18. See Chafete, J. S., and Dworkin, A. G., *Female Revolt: Women's Movements in World and Historical Perspective* (New Jersey: Rowmant Allaheld, 1986).

19. International Council of Women, *Women in a Changing World,* 3.

20. Ibid.

21. Minutes of Meeting at Buffalo, 1901, Typescript address. ICNA.

22. *British Journal of Nursing* (August 21, 1909): 151.

23. British Nurses Association, First Annual Report of the British Nurses Association (London, 1889).

24. See Anne Summers, *Angels and Citizens: British Women as Military Nurses, 1864–1914* (London: Routledge, 1988), 182–193, for a full discussion of this issue.

25. Second Quinquennial Meeting of the International Council of Nurses, 1909, 15. ICNA.

26. Ibid.

27. See Summers, *Angels and Citizens,* 277, for a full discussion of women's organizational response to the growing nationalist fervor surrounding the German military threat.

28. M. Meseurer, Director of Assistance Publique, Paris, Interim Conference of the International Council of Nurses, Paris, 1907, cited in Breay and Fenwick, 35 and 44.

29. Lavinia Dock, et al., *History of American Red Cross Nursing* (New York: The Macmillan Co., 1922), 75–93.

30. Ibid., 757.

31. Ibid., 757–759.

32. *Rapports de la Conference Internationale du Nursing, Paris, 1907* (Bordeaux, 1907), 8. [not only as a medical agent but an instrument of moral and social progress]. ICNA.

33. Second Quinquennial Meeting of the International Council of Nurses, 1909, 15. ICNA.

34. Fenwick Address, Second Quinquennial of the International Council of Nurses, 1909, cited in Breay and Fenwick, 47.

35. Ibid., 47.

36. Lavinia Dock, "Foreign Department: Items," *American Journal of Nursing,* 8 (April 1908): 539.

37. Lavinia Dock, "Foreign Department: International Reports Sent to Dowager Queen of Sweden," *American Journal of Nursing,* 10 (June 1910): 107–108.

38. Lavinia Dock, "The International Council and Congress in London," *American Journal of Nursing,* 9 (August 1909): 594.

39. Lavinia Dock, "Foreign Department: The Cologne Congress," *American Journal of Nursing,* 12 (August 1912): 656.

40. *British Journal of Nursing* (August 21, 1909): 151–153; Summers, *Angels and Citizens,* 275.

41. Lavinia Dock, "Foreign Department: The International Council of Nurses," *American Journal of Nursing*, 9 (July 1909): 508.
42. Breay and Fenwick, 60–67.
43. Ibid., 66.
44. Breay and Fenwick, 47.
45. Ibid.
46. Breay and Fenwick, 47.
47. Ibid. For an account of the fate of carriers of disease in the Progressive era, see Judith Walzer Leavitt, *Typhoid Mary—Captive to the Public's Health* (Boston: Beacon Press, 1996).
48. Breay and Fenwick, 47.
49. Ibid., 65.
50. Ibid.
51. Second Quinquennial Meeting, 1909, 77.
52. Lavinia Dock, *Hygiene and Morality* (New York: Putnam, 1910).
53. Dock, *Red Cross Nursing*, 1150–1152.
54. Breay and Fenwick, 47.
55. Second Quinquennial Meeting, 1909, 37–39.
56. Third Business Meeting of the International Council of Nurses, Cologne, 1912, "Text of Resolutions," 21. ICNA.
57. Second Quinquennial Meeting, 1909, 38.
58. Ibid., 38–39.
59. Ibid., 39.
60. C. Law, *Suffrage and Power: The Women's Movement, 1918–1928* (London: I. B. Tauns, 1997).
61. For a portrait of Edwardian feminism, see B. Harrison, *Prudent Revolutionaries* (Oxford and London: Oxford University Press, 1991) 1–16; *Second Annual Report of the Women's Social and Political Union, 1908* (London: The Women's Press, 1909); *Sixth Annual Report of the Women's Social and Political Union, 1914* (London: The Women's Press, 1915).
62. Lavinia Dock, "Foreign Department: The Cologne Congress," *American Journal of Nursing*, 12 (October 1912): 814.
63. Bridges, 45–46.
64. Lavinia Dock, "Foreign Department: The Progress of Women," *American Journal of Nursing*, 9 (November 1909): 842–845.
65. Breay and Fenwick, 97; "The International Council of Nurses," *British Journal of Nursing* (August 3, 1912): 93–94; Idem., (September 14, 1912): 200–202.
66. Breay and Fenwick, 93.
67. Third Business Meeting of the International Council of Nurses, Cologne, 1912, 22. ICNA.
68. Ibid.
69. Ibid., 23–49.
70. Third Regular Meeting, 24. ICNA.
71. Ibid., 37.
72. Ibid., 32.
73. See preceding chapter. Geertje Boschma, "Agnes Karll and the Creation of an Independent German Nursing Association, 1900–1927," *Nursing History Review*, 4 (1996): 151–168.

74. Lavinia Dock,"Foreign Department: Plans for the Cologne Conference," *American Journal of Nursing*, 11 (September 1911): 720–721; Idem., "The Eight-Hour System in New Zealand," *American Journal of Nursing*, 12 (May 1912): 414.

75. Lavinia Dock, "Foreign Department: The English Insurance Act," *American Journal of Nursing*, 13 (June 1913): 443.

76. Ibid.

77. H. Hecker, *The Overstrain of Nurses* (London, International Council of Nurses, 1912). Dr. Hecker's address to the Congress was translated and published as a pamphlet.

78. G. Cadbury, *Experiments in Industrial Organisation* (London: Longman, 1912).

79. See Paul Weindling (Ed.), *The Social History of Occupational Health* (London: Croom Helm, 1975), 12, for a discussion of the historical antecedents of debates on industrial health and efficiency.

80. Lavinia Dock, "Foreign Department: Old Age Insurance and Health Questions,"*American Journal of Nursing*, 9 (June 1909): 429–431; P. Wilson, "'The Golden Factory': Industrial Health and Scientific Management in an Italian Light Engineering Firm, The Magneti Marelli in the Fascist Period," in Paul Weindling (Ed.), *Occupational Health*, 240–257.

81. Dock attributed to Miss Nightingale suffragist sympathies—an idea derived from her reading of Cook's monumental biography. Sir Edward Cook, *The Life of Florence Nightingale* (London: Macmillan, 1913) 2 Vols. See Bridges, 46. Fenwick rationalized Miss Nightingale's lack of support for registration on the basis of her invalidism during the "first round" of politics. In fact, Miss Nightingale was working against registration behind the scenes from her bed, a campaign in which she was a central, albeit clandestine, contender.

82. Lavinia Dock, "Foreign Department: Official Announcements," *American Journal of Nursing*, 8 (October 1908): 701, 793.

83. "The Panama-Pacific Exposition," *British Journal of Nursing* (August 17, 1912): 129. Bridges, 43–48.

84. Breay and Fenwick, 91; "The International Council of Nurses," *British Journal of Nursing* (August 26, 1913): 327.

85. Bridges, 48.

86. Lavinia Dock, "Foreign Department: The War," *American Journal of Nursing*, 15 (February 1915): 136.

87. Letter from Miss Goodrich to Miss Breay, 17 April, 1915, cited in Breay and Fenwick, 113–114.

88. Ibid., 111. Florence Nightingale died in 1910.

89. "International News," *British Journal of Nursing* (September 26, 1914): 240.

90. Lavinia Dock, "Foreign Department: War Nursing Abroad," *American Journal of Nursing* 15 (March 1915): 497–499.

91. Ibid., 497.

92. Lavinia Dock, "Foreign Department: As to Preparedness," *American Journal of Nursing*, 16 (May 1916): 751–752.

93. Jeanne C. van Lanschot Hubrecht, "Foreign Department: A Letter from Holland," *American Journal of Nursing*, 17 (December 1916): 229–232.

94. Lavinia Dock, "Foreign Department," *American Journal of Nursing*, 15 (May 1915): 665–667; Idem., "The Holland Nurse's Association,"*American Journal of Nursing*, 18 (April 1918): 322.

95. Lavinia Dock, "Foreign Department," *American Journal of Nursing*, 19 (April 1919): 291.

96. Lavinia Dock, "Foreign Department: The International Congress," *American Journal of Nursing,* 15 (January 1915): 311–312.

97. Bridges, 50.

98. Bridges, 51–52.

99. Ibid., 118.

100. *The ICN,* 1 (1926): 75–76. ICNA.

101. Editorial, "The Spirit of Internationalism," *British Journal of Nursing,* XLIX (August 3, 1912): 83.

102. Lavinia Dock, "Foreign Department: Our International Prospects," *American Journal of Nursing,* 19 (October 1919): 781–782. Quotation is on 781.

103. Ibid., 781. Two representatives, Mrs. Williams and Miss Adah Samuels (Thoms), from the National Association of Colored Graduate Nurses in the United States also attended the 1912 meeting.

104. See Shula Marks, *Divided Sisterhood: Race, Class and Gender in the South African Nursing Profession* (New York: St. Martin's Press, 1994) for a discussion of the effects of apartheid in South Africa, and see Darlene Clark Hine, *Black Women in White: Racial Conflict and Cooperation in the Nursing Profession, 1890–1950* (Bloomington, IN: Indiana University Press, 1989) for race relations in American nursing.

105. "The Trained Nurses' Association of India," *American Journal of Nursing,* 12 (August 1912): 87. See the next chapter for more on this situation.

106. Ibid., 781.

107. Lavinia Dock reports in the *American Journal of Nursing* of June 1909 on some initial contacts with the women's movement in Russia.

108. *The ICN,* 1 (1926): 32–39. ICNA.

109. Ibid., 35.

110. See *American Journal of Nursing* of October 1909, 755–758 and see Huda Abu-Saad, *Nursing, A World View* (St. Louis: Mosby, 1979), 78–84.

111. Lavinia Dock, *American Journal of Nursing* (October 1909): 755–758. Quotation is on 756.

112. Abu-Saad, *A World View,* 78–83.

113. Ibid., 80.

114. Alexandra Romanoff, "Russian Nursing and Nurses. Part II," *The ICN,* 1 (1926): 117–123.

115. Ibid. See Abu-Saad (1979), 78–80. Having been a Red Cross nurse with the White Army, Romanoff's report is very negative about the Communist transformation.

116. Lavinia Dock, "Impressions of the Congress," *British Journal of Nursing* (August 24, 1912): 156.

117. Breay and Fenwick, 24.

118. Lavinia Dock, "Foreign Department: Letters from Denmark," *American Journal of Nursing* 16 (January, 1916): 58.

119. *The ICN,* Bulletin I (January 1924): 25–27; *The ICN,* Bulletin IV (October 1924): 49–50. The similarity in Scandinavian languages made the exchange easy to realize. Furthermore, the countries were politically closely related. Norway had even been part of Denmark for a long time.

120. Nete Balslev Wingender, *The Northern Nurses Federation 1920–1995* (Oslo, Norway: Northern Nurses Federation, 1995).

121. Breay and Fenwick, 125.

122. Sophie Nelson, "Foreign Department: International Council of Nurses, Informal Re-

port of the Fourth Regular Meeting, Copenhagen, Denmark," *American Journal of Nursing,* 22 (November 1922): 918–919.

123. Fourth Regular Meeting of the International Council of Nurses, Copenhagen, 1922, 128. ICNA.
124. Ibid., 130.
125. Anne Marie Rafferty, *The Politics of Nursing Knowledge* (London and New York: Routledge, 1996), 140–144.
126. Fourth Regular Meeting, 1922, 54–55.
127. Ibid., 132.
128. Ibid., 133.
129. Rafferty, *Politics,* 140–144.
130. Fourth Regular Meeting, 1922, 69.
131. Wingender, 3.
132. Fourth Regular Meeting, 1922, 58.
133. Ibid., 58–59.
134. Ibid., 59.
135. Treasurer Breay reported that at the end of the second quinquennial period (in 1909), the balance in hand of the ICN's account was £16.14s. Second Quinquennial Meeting, 1909, 18. ICNA. By 1912, the balance had increased to £44.00. See Report from Third Regular Meeting, 1912, 15. ICNA.
136. Report from Third Regular Meeting, 1912, 14.
137. Frontispiece, Second Quinquennial Meeting, 1909. ICNA.

# THREE

# Seeking Stability in the Midst of Change

*MERYN STUART*
*with Geertje Boschma*

$\mathcal{D}$uring the years between the end of World War I and the beginning of World War II, two problems preoccupied the International Council of Nurses (ICN) leadership: they had to keep the organization focused on its mission and they had to find new ways to function harmoniously. Throughout the period, they confronted pressing public health needs in many countries; potentially divisive racial, ethnic, economic, and class tensions among nations and nurses; and continued frustration in attaining shared international standards for nursing education. If all this were not enough, the ICN was also an organization with very low income, no permanent office, and changing presidential leadership every 3 years.

After the terrible losses, interruptions, and transitions of World War I, their first thought was to rebuild and expand the ICN's mission and membership. To do so, ICN leaders aimed to smooth over conflicts, reinforce commonalities among nurses, and broaden the organization's "international ideal." Again stressing commonality and unity among nurses, they sought to create a stable and collective whole, which, although representative of its parts, remained dedicated to preserving the overarching, essential idea of nursing. Continuity of leadership by like-minded people from Denmark, Finland, England, and the United States helped ensure the organization's survival during this time.

## The New Leadership

In 1922, after Lavinia Dock resigned, Denmark's Christiane Reimann assumed the position of honorary secretary. Reimann's appointment was important for three reasons. First, as the ICN struggled to maintain financial stability and increase membership after the war, Reimann's fluency in several languages enhanced international communication. Second, because Reimann was independently wealthy, she not only did not require a salary but regularly subsidized the ICN's limited coffers. Finally, Reimann's full-time secretarial status created informed continuity in the intervals between scheduled meetings of the ICN's elected officers and council.[1]

Finland's Baroness Sophie Mannerheim took over as ICN president, and Margaret Breay of Great Britain continued as treasurer. Before assuming her role as ICN president, Baroness Mannerheim headed the National Nurses' Association of Finland, founded in 1898, which was an early member of the ICN. Born in 1863, Mannerheim grew up on the family estate of Count Carl Robert Mannerheim and Helene von Julin. After a brief secretarial career and years traveling abroad, Mannerheim married Sir Hjalmar Linder. Their ill-fated marriage ended a short time later. Mannerheim entered nurse training at St. Thomas' Hospital in London and, upon graduation in 1902, worked in a sanatorium for scrofulous (tubercular) children. Two years later, she assumed matron responsibilities at a Helsinki surgical hospital. Using ideas from Florence Nightingale and with the support of the hospital's medical staff, Mannerheim reformed the nurse training system following the British model.[2]

The ascendancy of northern European nurses to presidential and secretarial positions—first in 1915 by Denmark's Henny Tscherning, then Finland's Sophie Mannerheim and Denmark's Christiane Reimann in 1922—introduced both new viewpoints and a dilution of British and American dominance in the leadership. For the first time since 1899, American and British nurses did not hold key leadership roles in the ICN.

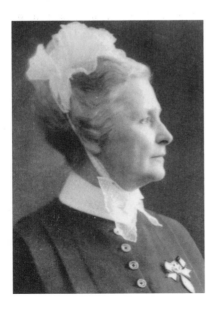

**FIGURE 3-1**
*Sophie Mannerheim, ICN President 1922 to 1925. From Bridges, A History of the International Council of Nurses, 1967.*

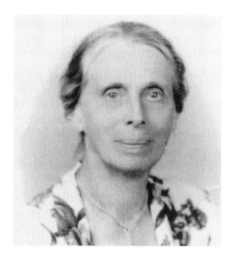

**FIGURE 3-2**
*Christiane Reimann, ICN's first Executive, 1922 to 1933. From Bridges, A History of the International Council of Nurses, 1967.*

At the same time, the Danish and Finnish nursing associations had a history of enduring relationships with earlier ICN activists. Indeed, Tscherning, Mannerheim, and Reimann all trained or practiced as nurses in either British or American systems. Shared cultural beliefs and friendship among the new and old leaders shored up the ICN's chances of finding what American Adelaide Nutting (who was actually a Canadian national) called the "best common working ground."

When Baroness Mannerheim officially took over the ICN presidency in 1923, there were fourteen affiliated national organizations: Great Britain, the United States, Germany, Canada, Denmark, Finland, Holland, India, New Zealand, Belgium, Italy, China, Norway, and South Africa. All representatives from these member nations were either Europeans or North Americans. The balance in the ICN treasury was a mere £110, partly because countries paid an affiliation fee rather than a per capita dues rate. The only way the ICN had managed to pay its bills, Breay noted in her Treasurer's Report, was through the generosity of Lavinia Dock and "an anonymous donor from Great Britain" (Margaret Breay herself). Dock donated the £90 royalty fee from volumes three and four of her *History of Nursing*. Ethel Gordon Fenwick provided 24 years of free space for ICN documents and records storage. By these means, the ICN retained its image as a "self supporting, self governing and therefore, self respecting body of professional workers."[3] These personal investments proved critical to a still new nurses' organization struggling to be independent and financially self-supporting.

But financial independence would be even more difficult in the postwar period, especially given the ICN's plans for expansion. The 1922 Grand Council Meeting decision to increase communication between member countries through publication of *The ICN*, for example, overwhelmed the organization's meager treasury. The new secretary, Christiane Reimann, ultimately paid the cost of *The ICN* herself because there was no budget for it.[4]

## The World After World War I

It seemed that everything was changed after the war. In a Round Table on Professional Ethics held at the 1925 Congress, the Danish Chair, Charlotte Munck, wrote that the new generation of nurses was different than the old—the conclusion of the group was that "the young generation cannot and will not submit to authority." Munck believed that the war, with all its excitement, its upheaval of the monotony of daily life, and its fearful experiences, created among many people (and certainly among nurses) a bitter distaste for daily routine duties, and a craving for excitement and new experiences that made it difficult for them to concentrate on their duties.[5]

Some ICN leaders reiterated the value of good feminine character, even giving it primacy over the importance of higher education. "A good nurse must be a good woman," France's Leonie Chaptal reiterated, "a very good woman, a born nurse."[6] Historian Mary Louise Roberts points out that in postwar France gender was a central metaphor in the cultural crisis. The horrors and devastation faced by the men (and some women) at the front reversed everything. Women worked in factories and entered the professions in unprecedented numbers while maintaining sole responsibility for their home while men were away at war. Gender boundaries were blurred, even erased. After the war, however, the older domestic ideal of the faithful, good, subservient woman in the home caring for men and children was reinvoked. Woman's "essential nature" reemerged with a vengeance. Pronatalism intensified after the war's slaughter; in France, even single women were encouraged to bear children. Motherhood and nurturing returned as the highest value in a woman's life.[7]

Still, other voices insisted on a new place for women. In the second *The ICN*, dated April 1924, Lavinia Dock's letter to "our members" is adamant about the role of women and nurses in the postwar world:

> The post war time we are in is one of change, fluctuation, growth undoubtedly—and also destruction, suffering, and even despair for great masses of people. Those who have always believed in the saving graces of human nature have perceived a special abundance of such redeeming and saving gifts in the woman of the race. We feminists, looking abroad over the earth, seeing the destructive and terrible results of unmodified male rule, are convinced that the only hope for civilization lies in the advance of women to places of power in the executive and administrative groups, which govern our world and control its destinies.

The ICN confronted the new political alliances and geographic boundaries, along with rampant destruction, hunger, poverty, and illness that characterized much of Europe and Russia. The countries actively overrun in the war were transformed, and others such as Canada, geographically remote from the fighting, would never be the same. Canadian author Sandra Gwyn later remarked that it was "the Great War that mark[ed] the real birth of Canada" rather than the 1867 Confederation of four British colonies. "The effort of mobilizing and equipping a vast army," she claimed, "modernized us, and our blood and our accomplishments transformed us from colony to nation."[8]

In historian E. H. Carr's somewhat ironic perspective, the postwar period was,

> [a] golden age of continuously expanding territories and markets, of a world policed by the self-assured and not too onerous British hegemony . . . of the easy assumptions that what was good for one was good for all and that what was economically right could not be morally wrong, . . . for some, it was a time of hope and economic renewal.[9]

Hope and renewal for some shared the stage with intense nationalism, as conflict between richer nations and poorer states suffused the international arena.[10] New states and new political parties were forming throughout Europe and the Far East. Political revolutions were starting again in China and ending in Russia.

The nurses of Germany and Russia were stark examples of individuals immersed in political unrest or revolution, homelessness, and even starvation. Germany, forced by the Treaty of Versailles to pay huge amounts of postwar reparation, found its economy devastated, resulting in high inflation and high unemployment.[11] The Professional Organization of German Nurses (*Berufsorganisation der Krankenpflegerinnen Deutschlands*) was financially destitute and barely able to maintain itself. Unemployment among German nurses was rampant. Many, according to Karll, lost their homes, their livelihoods and their lives. Nurses' status, vividly described by Karll in her "Report on Nursing in Germany," worsened considerably after the French and Belgian occupation of the Ruhr area in 1923.

> The nurses endure probably twice or three times as much as people of other professions, because they in their work are witnesses of the greatest human sufferings and grief. It is no wonder that there is a growing number of suicides even among the nurses. A short time ago a most sympathetic nurse, who was engaged in social work took her own life. The Doctor gave us as a cause: failing health combined with the mental pressure of not being able to assist others enough. I am sure it is of the greatest help for most of us to belong to an organization where we can come together and meet for full understanding.[12]

Karll highlighted the ICN's importance in sustaining German nurses' morale, noting that without help received from friends abroad, the German Nurses Organization would have disappeared altogether. Indeed, ICN Secretary Christiane Reimann had asked member associations to send money and clothing to Germany; 150 disabled and impoverished German nurses received food and clothing. In spite of moral and fiscal support from the ICN, however, the situation in Germany and among German nurses remained bleak. Later in 1924, with her own physical health failing after a mastectomy and radiation therapy, Karll explained the plight of nurses working in hospitals to readers of *The ICN*:

> Curious [sic] enough they get in the Berlin Hospital only supper on *two days* a week and are told they had a loaf of bread and margarine for the other two days. But this is so little that they could not eat more than two very thin slices for supper . . . the nurses keep all the remains of dinner for the pupil nurses but they begin after a short time to fail in health.[13]

In Russia, similar chaos and dislocation prevailed. When the White Army of the czar left Crimea in 1920, approximately 1500 formally trained Red Cross nurses fled the country along with sick and wounded soldiers. Leaving home with only their uniforms on their backs, the nurses became refugees throughout Europe. Though retrained by National Red Cross Societies in Turkey, Serbia, Bulgaria and Belgium, many nurse refugees were unable to find nursing work and instead went into factory, office, bank and domestic service. Refugee nurses, according to Russian correspondent Alexandria Romanoff, were "victims of an overwhelming catastrophe that has reversed normal conditions," while those who remained in Russia witnessed the "complete destruction" of previously known political, social, and economic institutions."[14] Russian nurses did seek and receive aid from the ICN. As Romanoff put it, "Russian nurses appreciate immensely this truly sisterly attitude toward them and this feeling of fellowship with colleagues in other countries will sustain and comfort them."[15]

In exile, nursing leaders of the Russian Red Cross attempted to reestablish an organization for Russian refugee nurses.[16] Alexandra Romanoff, who was director of nursing services of the deposed Russian Red Cross founded the Union of Russian Nurses Abroad in 1922 in an attempt to reunite the refugee nurses scattered in Serbia, Bulgaria, and Turkey.[17] However, given the insurmountable political barriers, nurses remaining in Russia were never able to join their professional colleagues in the ICN. Like their German sisters, Russian nurses faced dismal times. The 1917 October Revolution marked the beginning of ultimate government takeover by the Communist Party and, with it, dramatic changes in Russian medical and nursing services. As noted in the preceding chapter, nurses, like other workers, were required to join unions but were forbidden to strike or bargain for better working conditions. Hospital and public health reform efforts initiated in the pre-Revolution period stopped. By 1921, Communist Party schools of nursing reopened with new and different professional standards and curricula. During the 1920s, a few accounts of health conditions and nursing affairs in Russia were circulated by visitors from other countries. The redoubtable Quaker Anna Haines, for instance, who visited Russia several times on behalf of the American Friends Service Committee, offered Westerners some idea of the Russian Commissariat of Health and its nationalized health system.[18] But, for all intents and purposes, Russian nurses remained cut off from their professional colleagues in the West until the Iron Curtain fell more than 50 years later.

## New ICN Agendas

When the first postwar Grand Council meeting in 1922 convened in Copenhagen, Danish nurse Henny Tscherning, president of the ICN since 1915, was finally able to relinquish the office to Baroness Mannerheim. Due to problems of travel and the low rate of monetary exchange, however, only ten representatives of national nurses organizations attended the council.[19] Nonetheless, several proposed resolutions reveal the concerns of the ICN leadership. Among these was a resolution defining the standard for nurse training as a "three year program taught by professional nurses." At a time when "the Council was battling for its existence and having to prove its usefulness or disappear," the ICN was trying to universalize a standard for nurse training that would be shared across the nursing world.[20] The following year, in August 1923, a special meeting of the executive committee and an informal conference sponsored by the ICN raised other important issues. At the conference, Christiane Reimann informed members that "important issues are to be considered and possibly a thorough change of the policy held up till now."[21] Thirty-three women from Great Britain, the United States, Finland, New Zealand, Bulgaria, France, Iceland, Poland, Romania, and Serbia attended the special meeting. Many participants were American and British expatriots who were starting nursing schools in eastern Europe.

On the packed agenda were important questions: a possible collaboration with the nursing division of the League of Red Cross Societies (LRCS), the ICN's relationship with the newly formed European Council for Nursing Education (ECNE), the need for a functioning ICN headquarters, and, perhaps most worrisome, the British College of Nursing's bid for ICN membership. Great Britain, was, of course, already represented by the National Council of Trained Nurses of Great Britain and Ireland led by Fenwick.

# The ICN and the LRCS

Many countries used quickly trained Red Cross "nurses" during the war as readily available and inexpensive adjuncts to their limited cadres of professional nurses. In some countries, war-trained military nurses continued to be treated as fully qualified professional nurses after the war. For example, the British nursing establishment struggled with what to do with 50,000 Voluntary Aid Detachment workers (VADs). Britain's professional nurses feared that VADs might claim equal status to trained nurses after their war service.[22]

Dock had been particularly percipient in worrying that the Red Cross would try to organize a peacetime nursing service.[23] The possibility of Red Cross involvement, not only in peacetime nursing but also public health activities, filled Dock with horror. She quickly saw the threat of the ICN being eclipsed by the Red Cross and public health nurses absorbed within the hierarchical structure of the much larger international organization.[24] By 1921, however, Dock seemed to have changed her mind, presumably pacified by the knowledge that the LRCS and their courses in international public health in London were being overseen by the American nurse, Alice Fitzgerald.[25] Indeed, the fact that the LRCS was something of an American invention, heavily influenced by the American Red Cross, may have helped to allay Dock's worst fears.

Although Baroness Mannerheim wanted to build and maintain good relations between the LRCS and the ICN, she vigorously defended the value of trained over untrained nurses, whether in times of war or peace. The LRCS was anxious to move ahead with solving nurse shortage problems in Europe and seemed less concerned with how fully prepared some of its nurses might be.

Mannerheim fought against certifying women as nurses after only a few weeks or months of training and protested positioning the lesser trained practitioners in charge of fully trained nurses. She argued that this practice ultimately damaged the professional identity of fully trained nurses, who, she argued, should be in charge of war relief work.

Bending to Mannerheim's persistence and pressure, the LRCS appointed an Advisory Board of Nursing to advise it on nursing matters. Consisting of six professional nurses, of whom four were active ICN members, the board advised the league to stop titling women "Red Cross Nurses" after they completed short courses of instruction. Instead, the new trainees would be called Voluntary Aid Detachments and serve under fully trained Red Cross nurses. The board further recommended that the League desist from creating national professional nursing organizations that, by their composition, were unable to affiliate with the ICN. This latter move helped strengthen the ICN's position as nursing's international voice for education and practice standards. The ICN leadership, keen to represent nurses worldwide in matters of the public's health, hoped to expand on this success.[26]

## Continuing the Public Health Agenda

Indeed, the essential importance of improving public health was one of the most discussed topics in ICN's journal in the 1920s and 1930s, especially after 1925. American public health leader, Mary Gardner, wrote in 1926 that "money was never more plentiful for all forms of health work than during and directly succeeding the war years, nor was public opinion ever so ready to back excursions into the field of experimentation."[27]

Money for public health practice and education came primarily from the LRCS, the League of Nations's Health section, more affluent nations, and private philanthropic foundations, especially the Rockefeller Foundation. Nurses came to be seen as the ideal front-line workers in this new postwar reform.[28]

In 1920, the LRCS initiated and supported an international course for public health nurses at King's College, London, England, later moving to Bedford College. American nurses Alice Fitzgerald and Katherine Olmsted served as the first and second directors of the new program. Through lectures, conferences, individual field demonstrations and "excursions," international course leaders aimed to "prepare qualified nurses for executive and teaching positions in connection with health activities such as visiting nursing, infant welfare and child conservation work, school nursing, tuberculosis nursing, and nursing under municipal, state or Red Cross authorities." By 1924, 51 students from 34 countries and sponsored in a variety of ways had taken the course.[29] Nurses were also sent to Yale University in the United States and to the University of Toronto, Canada for public health training.

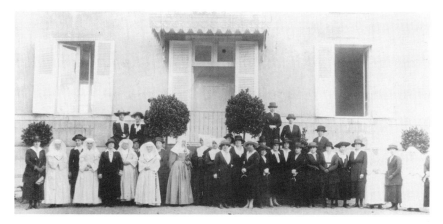

FIGURE 3-3
*The Congress at Nantes—a group of Health Visitors, 1924. Courtesy of the Rockefeller Archive Center.*

Between 1923 and 1925, Sophie Mannerheim, Katherine Olmsted, the new LRCS director of nursing, and Sir Claude Hill, director general of the LRCS, corresponded regularly. Their letters reveal the competition and conflict between the ICN and the League that Mannerheim attempted to remedy. The ICN and the League differed about who could, or should, speak for nursing in the international community.[30] Mannerheim, Olmsted, and Hill also disagreed about who could be called a nurse, about standards for schools of nursing, who should set them, about laypersons and physicians having power over nursing decisions, and about whether Red Cross nurses should join separate nursing organizations or affiliate with the ICN.

In 1924, during the first LRCS Nursing Advisory Board Meeting, for example, Hill argued that advisory board recommendations might be impossible to carry out because the League "was not a nursing association but an organization which one might almost say was trying to make bricks out of straw." No matter how much the League believed in the "highest development of nursing throughout the world," he continued, it was essentially a "servant" of the National Red Cross Societies.[31] Despite these extensive and basic ideologic disagreements, Mannerheim created good relations with Hill and Olmsted and later chaired the nursing advisory committee of the League, against the wishes of many American nurses and other nursing colleagues. Adelaide Nutting and Isabel Stewart, for example, warned Mannerheim against associating with Olmsted, who they viewed as out of touch with international nursing. As Nutting put it,

> Miss Olmsted is young, ardent and very well-meaning, but her complete unfamiliarity with the International Council of Nurses, its history and, in fact, its actual reasons for existence make it difficult for her to envisage in any adequate way the nursing problem in Europe.[32]

The threat to the ICN by the LRCS Division of Nursing, under Olmsted's direction, did worry Mannerheim. Throughout the 3 years of her presidency, the relationship between the LRCS and the ICN was the focus of many letters between Mannerheim and her confidantes in the United States. She regularly sought advice from Clara Noyes, Elizabeth Fox, Isabel Stewart, and Adelaide Nutting about problems facing international nursing, particularly as related to the politics in British nursing and the LRCS.

Although she chose to keep her ties with Olmsted and Hill, Mannerheim remained steadfast in her opinion that the ICN, not the League, bore responsibility for setting worldwide nursing standards. Her success at negotiating this delicate ground was measured when, later, it was Mannerheim who was asked to replace Olmsted when she resigned as director of the LRCS Nursing Division in 1926.[33]

## More Conflict

Mannerheim's anxiety over the LRCS was matched only by her concern about the creation of the ECNE. Mannerheim thought the organization's nurse founders were intent on establishing another potentially divisive organization instead of joining the ICN. Mannerheim believed nonmember European countries needed the ICN's help to improve their 2-year nurse training programs. But Enid Newton, who founded a nursing school in Serbia, replied that many European nurses were reluctant to seek the ICN's assistance because they believed they could never meet the ICN's 3-year training standard. Most of the schools required 2 or less years of nurse training. To reconcile the goals of the two organizations, the ICN granted ECNE nurses honorary vice president positions on the ICN Council until their countries could form their own national associations made up of eligible nurses.

In another potentially divisive move, the British College of Nursing (founded in 1916) sought to affiliate with the ICN. Their request created another multifactorial and vexing problem. First, the college's board of directors included members who were not nurses; its constitution was, therefore, out of harmony with the ICN requirement for an all-nurse board. Second, the college's bid for admission raised the larger question of what to do when two or more nurses organizations from one country sought ICN affiliation. Fenwick viewed The National Council of Trained Nurses of Great Britain and Ireland as the "accredited channel through which relations can be established with the ICN."[34] She vehemently opposed

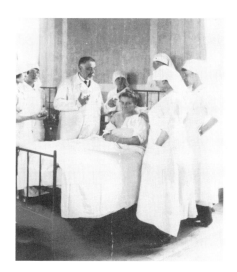

**FIGURE 3-4**
*School for Health Visitors in France, 1924. Courtesy of the Rockefeller Archive Center.*

the prospect of another organization, hostile to her own, seeking and winning affiliation with the ICN.[35]

On this matter, Mannerheim regularly corresponded with British nurse Alicia Lloyd Still and her assistant, Miss Coode. Communication centered on the "College of Nursing dilemma" and strategies aimed to bring the college, the largest representative of British nurses, into ICN ranks. Although Fenwick, as founder of the rival association, led the battle against the college's admission, there is no record of personal correspondence between Mannerheim and Fenwick about this matter.[36]

Fenwick's determined stance against the admission of two national associations into ICN membership differed from Mannerheim's more inclusive position. Mannerheim was willing to consider admission of two or more associations from one country in part because, in her own country, 300 Finnish-speaking nationalists broke away from the Swedish-speaking Association of Nurses in Finland to form a separate association. Although she found the division of Finnish nurses terribly sad, she confided to Vice President Clara Noyes in April 1925:

> As to my own point of view; it has not changed in the least since our association split into two by the separation of a large portion of the Finnish-speaking nurses . . . I should be entirely in favor of their becoming members of the International Council with exactly the same rights as ourselves. I do not yet see that there would be any danger about this, either in the case of Finland or of Great Britain.[37]

Mannerheim feared that if the ICN did not expand its eligibility criteria to admit "less than professional" nurses' associations, and at least consider more than one national association per country, the quiescent ECNE might reactivate. More inclusive of different types of nurses and organizations, the ECNE, led by France's Mlle. Chaptal, could, if it chose, directly compete with the ICN for members. Using exclusion rather than inclusion as a mechanism for admission, Mannerheim thought, could ultimately threaten the ICN's survival. In 1925, Mannerheim wrote Clara Noyes describing the ECNE's attitude. "They think," she wrote, "[that] the International Council [of Nurses] is simply an organization of American and Scandinavian nurses, and that the rest of Europe—taking no account of Germany, of course—is left outside, i.e. England, France, and the middle, east, and south of Europe."[38] Ultimately, Mannerheim's fears were alleviated when France applied for, and was accepted into ICN membership in 1925, along with Poland, Bulgaria, Cuba, and the Irish Free State.

Interestingly, France's admission followed the resignation of its longtime honorary vice president, Dr. Anna Hamilton, who served in that capacity from 1900 to 1925. A physician, naturalized French citizen, and Protestant, Hamilton wrote a 500-page thesis on hospital nursing for her French medical diploma in 1900. She later headed a Protestant hospital

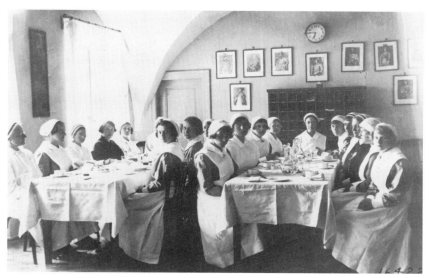

**FIGURE 3-5**
*School of Nursing, Cracow, Poland, 1926. Courtesy of the Rockefeller Archive Center.*

in Bordeaux and became the school's director. She eventually upgraded the school to a 3-year program and, in 1916, renamed it *Ecole Florence Nightingale*. Hamilton received generous postwar financial support from American nurses as well as Rockefeller Foundation funding for a public health dispensary, a new hospital, and a nurses' residence. Anna Hamilton died in the mid 1930s.

## A More Representative and Responsive Organization

In 1925, addressing these concerns about competition from without and division within, the ICN constitution was revised to reform ICN membership and organizational structure guidelines. Written by American Clara Noyes, it was the first revision since 1900; its broad outlines brought significant changes. First, a board of directors replaced the executive committee. The new board consisted of past presidents, the elected president, first and second vice presidents, treasurer, secretary, and the president elect from each member association. In countries without official ICN affiliation, voting associate national representatives could be appointed by the board of directors. Future congresses would be held every 4 years rather than every 3 years.[39]

Members were reclassified as either active or honorary. Active status meant that only *one* national nurse association per country, composed of trained nurses, could serve as the official council member. Not coincidentally, the new definition followed on the heels of the British College of Nursing's affiliation with Fenwick's National Council of Trained Nurses in order to officially associate with the ICN. The consolidation of the two British professional associations solved, for the moment, the problem created for ICN when competing interests arise among nurses in their own countries.

To forestall rival organizations (such as the ECNE) from signing up countries whose nurse associations were either unorganized or unable to meet ICN membership standards, the ICN created the honorary associate national representative category. Although their countries could not officially vote in matters of ICN policy and practice, associate national representatives were given limited voting power on the grand council.

Once membership policy was reformed, the ICN board members turned their attention to the ICN's financial and structural integrity. Annual dues for active member associations were increased to 5 American cents *per capita* or the equivalent currency of the country. Having secured increased income, the ICN next focused on ways to decrease spending. The costly journal, for example, was to become self-supporting, paid for by individual subscriptions rather than out of general funds.

It was also decided that Geneva, Switzerland would become the permanent headquarters of the ICN, partly because Reimann favored Switzerland's neutral political status and partly because of the country's stable economy. Reimann, who was both a board member and now executive secretary, was increasingly influential in council business decisions. She communicated and visited regularly with leaders in nursing and other international organizations. Her letters to Mannerheim in preparation for the congress suggest that Reimann frequently made independent decisions, gave advice freely, and offered forceful opinions on any subject concerning the ICN, its leaders, or its members.

In 1927, an interim conference and board of directors meeting were held in Geneva. The new ICN president, American Nina Gage, founder and dean of the Hunan-Yale School of Nursing in Peking and representing China, presided over the meeting. Gage was founding president of the Chinese National Association of Nurses (NAC) before her election to ICN presidency in 1925. England's Ellen Musson succeeded Margaret Breay as treasurer, a position she would hold until 1947.

The 1927 board of directors meeting focused on Musson's treasurer's report as well as on Reimann's extensive secretary's report. Reimann was recognized for her "almost superhuman piece of work" between 1925 and 1927 during which she had visited 20 countries, edited the journal, opened and furnished the new office in Geneva, corresponded regularly with all member associations, met with many international organizations, started

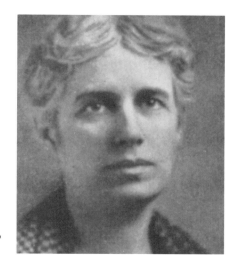

**FIGURE 3-6**
*Nina Gage, ICN President 1925 to 1929. From AJN Collection.*

a library, and hired two assistants. She augmented the salary of one of the assistants from her own personal funds.[40]

Indeed, Reimann habitually spent her own money to clear deficits of various ICN projects. This was an uncomfortable, even unpalatable situation for some board members who felt ambivalent about Reimann's role. Because of slow reimbursement, Reimann asked at this meeting that funds for the journal be managed through ICN headquarters rather than out of the treasurer's office in England. Both Treasurer Musson and Fenwick refused Reimann's request, even though they continued to welcome her

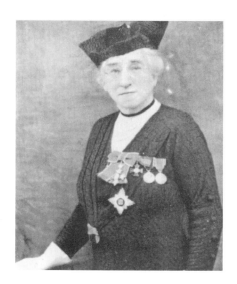

**FIGURE 3-7**
*Ellen Musson of Great Britain, ICN Treasurer 1925 to 1947. From Bridges, A History of the International Council of Nurses, 1967.*

financial support. The ICN was plagued by cumbersome procedures and by fluctuating currency values in France and elsewhere.

## Facing East—China

The new ICN president, Nina Diadamia Gage (1883–1946), graduated from Wellesley College in Massachusetts in 1905 and the Roosevelt Hospital School of Nursing in New York City in 1908. Gage went to China in 1909 and remained there with only brief interruptions until 1927.

The situation in China, which would be transformed into a Communist republic in 1949, brought the ICN a new perspective on international nursing. Although trade relationships between Western countries and China existed from the 13th century, it was during the 19th century that Christian missions opened there. Elizabeth McKechnie, a graduate of the Woman's Hospital of Philadelphia, was the first Western trained nurse to go to China. In 1884, she joined Elizabeth Reifsnyder, a surgeon; together, they ran a small dispensary in Shanghai near West Gate.[41] According to missionary sources, 33 British and 41 Americans were working in China by 1887.[42] As time went on, Western imperialist politics dominated Chinese life. By 1900, Western countries (England, France, Russia, and the United States) divided control of China among themselves.

Western style universities and professional education began to develop in China in the early 20th century. Until then, education was based on Confucian traditions, which traditionally denied schooling to Chinese women. Although Western Protestant missions established some boarding schools for girls in the 19th century, it was not until after the 1911 revolution that lower and middle schools became coeducational. The pool of women from which nurses might be educated was, therefore, very small.[43] Many Chinese men who assimilated with the foreign powers sought education in western Europe or the United States.

Resistance grew among more educated Chinese people against the traditional political system in China. By 1911, nationalist revolutionists under the leadership of Sun Yat-sen established a Chinese republic. Western countries supported these attempts, although Western powers' conflicting interests complicated their imperialist politics. For example, Russia supported the growing Communist forces in China and helped to establish a Chinese Communist party in 1921. These tense relationships between nationalist, Communist and Western forces flared up in many civil wars in China during the 1920s and 1930s.

This turbulent political scene was the remarkable context for a flourishing Western health care system developed by foreign powers in China after the turn of the century. In the conservative province of Hunan, which opened up to foreigners in 1902 after the Boxer Movement revolts,

Western missions began opening hospitals. In 1906, for example, the American Yale mission opened a hospital in which the nursing initially was done by native Chinese servants.[44]

Seven years later, the provincial government and the Yale mission negotiated a plan to establish medical and nursing education. The government agreed to finance medical and nursing education for Chinese students and the Yale mission would staff the schools and hospital. This endeavor evolved into the Hunan-Yale University Medicine and Nursing Schools, which developed in close connection with the College of Yale in China.[45] The combined nursing and college courses led to a baccalaureate degree; a 3-year diploma training for nurses was offered as well. Both foreigners and Chinese students from upper-class families applied for the new education.

Because, according to Chinese customs, women could not take care of any men outside their families, men were sought for nursing education in the Hunan-Yale School. A separate educational system for men and women students was established. Similarly, the nursing school of the London Mission Men's Hospital, opened by two British nursing sisters in 1914, was solely for men. These Western-style training schools were on a small scale compared to the size of China. But, by the early 1920s, there were about 90 registered schools with 1600 nursing students including equal numbers of men and women. Many of these schools were supported by American and European philanthropic organizations.

The American Rockefeller Foundation, which developed a worldwide program to fight tuberculosis and other contagious diseases after World War I, was active in China. Between 1915 and 1947, it invested over $45 million there to aid government or university schools to train health personnel, particularly in public health and health administration.[46] In an early move, the foundation took over a medical mission in Peking, which later became the Peking Union Medical College (PUMC), connected with the Yenching University in Peking. In 1920, it opened a School of Nursing with American Anna D. Wolf as dean, succeeded in 1925 by Ruth Ingram, a graduate of the University of Pennsylvania Hospital Training School and Teacher's College, Columbia University. Following the new American university model, both a 3-year diploma training program and a 5-year combined college and nursing course leading to a baccalaureate were offered. High admission standards requiring middle school (high school) and English competency resulted in a low number of students. All teaching was in English after the school determined that English was a superior language for teaching modern science and medicine; this position caused controversy until PUMC finally rescinded it decades later.[47]

With the support of the China Medical Board, textbooks were translated and published in Chinese. By 1926, with the exception of PUMC, Chinese was the language of instruction in all schools. During these first decades, Chinese graduates remained subordinate to the foreign graduates; Chinese graduates were often appointed as auxiliaries and a distinction in title was made between native nurses and foreign graduates.[48] Chinese nurses accounted for two thirds of NAC's 1200 members by 1926, however, and a Chinese nurse was elected vice president.[49]

## The National Association of Nurses

The European and American nurses who led these foreign-dominated schools soon developed a Chinese national nursing organization. In 1914, at the first National Conference of nurses in Shanghai, a Chinese word for "nurse" was adopted, because no such word existed. Depending on local conditions, schools of nursing sometimes provided high school education along with nurse training.[50] By 1922, the NAC was holding biennial conferences. At first, most of the leadership of the 132-member association were foreign nurses. During the 1922 conference, a Committee on Nursing Education was established to regulate the training and registration of nursing schools with Nina Gage, Dean of the Hunan-Yale School of Nursing, as chair. The association gained control over professional standards because it successfully campaigned to make its own Committee on Nursing Education responsible for the examination of nurses.[51]

Familiarity between ICN leaders and the Western nurse leaders of the NAC eased acceptance into the ICN. In 1922, the NAC was admitted to the ICN at the fourth regular meeting in Copenhagen, Denmark, even though they sent no delegates to the meeting. The Chinese papers at this conference were read by the conference chairman, who acted as delegate pro tem.[52] The rapidly growing Chinese association was first represented by delegates at the 1925 ICN Conference in Helsinki, where Nina Gage immediately was elected as the seventh president of the ICN.

## Civil War in China

But, at about the same time, the political situation in China deteriorated, deeply interfering with the educational system established by the Western powers. In the southern province of Hunan, Communist groups were in power; they controlled the local government and organized laborers and students into unions. The unions, which demanded government by committee with student and labor representation, threatened the establishment to the point that all schools and hospitals in the area were closed or turned over to the so-called red government. By 1925, Nina Gage's letters to Yale reflected her discouragement.

> . . . parades are going on at the behest of the Union. And then they talk about "Imperialism" . . . . Our servants are all in the union . . . . They

demanded more wages, and refuse to let us dismiss anyone and manage with fewer servants than we had. So of course we cannot hold out long, but must go . . . .[53]

In the ICN journal of 1927, on her way home to the United States, Gage sadly reported the closing of the College of Yale in China, including the medical and nursing school. Students and faculty were scattered, and many foreigners returned to their countries of origin. The Peking Union School, however, continued to function under Chinese nurse leadership until 1953. Civil war continued until 1934 when the Communists were expelled from the south. After a short period of renewed cooperation between Nationalists and Communists when the Japanese invaded China, the Nationalist Party was defeated by the Communists and withdrew to Taiwan (Formosa) after World War II.

## Persistent Issues at the ICN

The 1929 Quinquennial Congress met in Montreal, Canada when the armed conflict and revolution in China interfered with the original plan to hold the congress there. Although over 6000 nurses from 38 countries attended the conference, 5000 were either Canadian or American. In her presidential address, Gage listed issues still on the ICN agenda after 30 years: the definition of "the trained nurse," the need for state registration and local and national organizations, communication through professional journals, the necessary preparation for military ("army") nursing, and uniform requirements and curricula for schools of nursing. Other topics on the agenda for over a decade included standardization of practice, "job analysis," work efficiency, numbers and types of nurses, and places of nurse employment.

Gage viewed Secretary Reimann as a key instrument for gathering needed data for many of the ICN's topics of concern. Appealing to the audience to support Reimann's secretarial duties, she claimed Reimann could make many interesting studies and help the profession greatly by her research, if she could be freed from some of her routine office duties.

In other words, Gage saw research about nurses and nursing as one of the ICN's key functions for the next decade. Because both Gage and Reimann had studied at Teacher's College, Columbia University, they were indoctrinated with Adelaide Nutting's and Isabel Stewart's beliefs about linking the art of nursing to a scientific base. By doing so, they argued, science could be harnessed to social reform; nursing could become more scientific without sacrificing its art and its humane functions.[54]

In her keynote speech, read by Elizabeth Burgess to the congress, impressively entitled "The Future," Adelaide Nutting also called for changes in the educational foundation and character of nursing as neces-

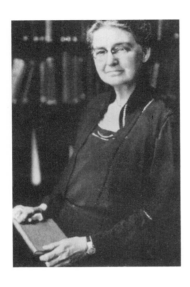

**FIGURE 3-8**
*Adelaide Nutting (USA). From AJN Collection.*

sary precursors to a successful future for nursing. One of the ways to achieve this future, she argued, was to develop and enforce nursing standards immune to hospital control.[55] Nutting, Annie Goodrich and Rebecca Thorogood Strong of Scotland all returned again and again to the incongruity of trying to establish science-based curricula outside of institutions of higher learning.[56]

Back in 1922, several important resolutions passed at the Grand Council meeting set forth the leadership's views with regard to acceptable nursing education. These were:

- [the] standard for trained professional women shall be three years continuous training in recognised, qualified training schools
- the training school be under the direction of a trained professional Nurse Superintendent
- the "Standard Curriculum" to be given under the direction of a professional nurse
- State registration and recognition be urged upon those National Councils in the countries where it is not already in force

By 1925, the ICN's Committee on Education was reorganized and enlarged to include a representative appointed by each of the 19 active member associations of the council as well as the 11 associate countries. Isabel Stewart took over the chair from Adelaide Nutting. After 1925, the emphasis was on helping countries implement the standard 3-year training program by publishing fundamental principles in constructing a curriculum.

In 1929, reporting as chair of the Nursing Education Committee, Isabel Stewart elaborated on ways to construct new nursing curriculums that emphasized optimum rather than minimum standards for nursing education and practice. The product of the committee's work, a 28-page report, appeared in 1930 after being presented to the 1929 Montreal Congress and getting feedback from 16 of 19 member countries.

In its Introduction, Stewart stressed nursing's commonality: "the astonishing thing is that there should be such a large measure of agreement on those principles which are most fundamental." By 1933, Stewart proudly reported, "the full report was issued . . . in seven different languages—English, French, German, Finnish, Spanish, Chinese and Dutch."[57]

However, Stewart was clearly aware of cultural differences and potential pitfalls and conflict around standardization. She began the report by saying it was a guide, not a law, and that the committee was "very opposed to the idea of a rigid and static curriculum, believing that no one pattern can be made to fit the needs of every school, in every country" (p. 7). She did assert, however, that since "the needs of human beings are much the same the world over" and that students should "be prepared to perform much the same kind of functions . . . there are certain fundamental principles of nursing and of education which should be incorporated into *every* nursing school curriculum." This last statement conformed to long-held beliefs that the ICN's "larger aims" should be kept before nurses of the world and that schools "should be helped to advance as rapidly as possible toward them." The report then detailed in 20, single-spaced pages just what the larger aims should be, including specific duties and responsibilities of professional nurses, facilities that should be used, staffing, work hours, and so forth. Certain Anglo-American cultural norms inhabited the report (eg, that nurses must be prepared to care for both sexes and all races and classes [p. 10] and that "definite guidance in the best use of leisure" should be part of education [p. 16]). Certain standards suggested by the committee would be very difficult to meet in many countries (eg, that training should occur in a large hospital with access to all kinds of "active" [as opposed to chronic] patients with medical, surgical, obstetric, and mental problems). Students should work only an 8-hour day, and should have limited night duty, individual residence rooms, quiet comfortable classrooms, and adequate laboratories. Moreover, Stewart firmly asserted that adequate training for nursing must include extensive practice under hospital conditions with responsible nurse directors, teachers, and supervisors.

## Money and Membership

The 1929 Congress still faced the precarious condition of the ICN budget plus the ongoing need for a full-time editor for its professional journal. On learning of their reliance on Reimann's purse and still fearing interference from more affluent, outside organizations like the LRCS, members raised annual per capita dues from 5 to 8 American cents. The Grand

Council believed their continuing dependence on personal donations from members lowered the organization's self-respect.

New members in 1929 included Sweden, the Philippines, Greece, Brazil, and Yugoslavia. The Korean Nurses Association (represented by Miss Shepping) applied for membership but was turned down because Korea, at that time, was under the domination of Japan. In effect, the ICN Membership Committee, after much discussion back and forth, accepted the view of the League of Nations (ie, that Japan did represent Korea). Again, the ICN struggled with unanticipated issues stemming from its rule that only one organization from each country could be considered. The Italian Nurses Association, a member since 1922, had ceased to exist under the Mussolini government. It was formally removed from the ICN list of members. At the same meeting, the application of the Fascist Association of Nurses of Italy was rejected with little debate.

A significant conflict developed over a motion by the Belgian nurses to restrict the leadership of national associations to native-born nurses, which would apply mostly in countries where nursing schools were founded and led by American and British nurses. This must have been somewhat awkward because the departing president of the ICN, Nina Gage, fit the definition of a foreigner who had led a national association (China). Secretary Reimann, who had raised this issue before, supported the motion to require native-born representatives saying, "I know that while some nurses have done splendid work in foreign countries, the native nurses very often

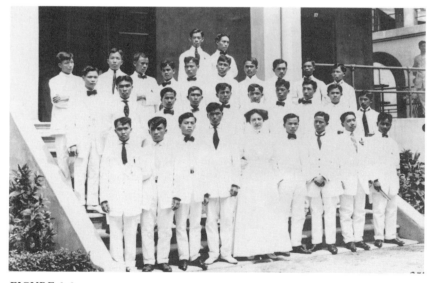

**FIGURE 3-9**
*Nurses at the Philippines General Hospital, 1929. Courtesy of the Rockefeller Archive Center.*

wish they would disappear . . . because they want to be independent." Those opposed to the motion, including Great Britain's Musson, argued that restricting leadership to nurses native to the country would lead to a situation in which it would be nearly impossible to find "women sufficiently educated and capable of assuming authority."[58] Despite strong support by Reimann and others, including the Canadian and Belgian representatives, the motion was soundly defeated.

## New Stability for the ICN

By 1931, the ICN represented 160,000 nurses, with 23 countries in affiliation. The business of the council kept Reimann and two assistants busy full time. They translated the journal into French and English and corresponded with member associations in ten languages.[59] With Leonie Chaptal of France now serving as president and the United States' Clara Noyes continuing as first vice president, the ICN looked increasingly more stable and able to manage its affairs.

Leonie Marie Chaptal was born in 1873, in Paris, France; her father's family was well known for political and scientific accomplishments whereas her mother's family were affluent bankers. Mlle. Chaptal was sickly as a child and was educated at home. Brought up as a Roman Catho-

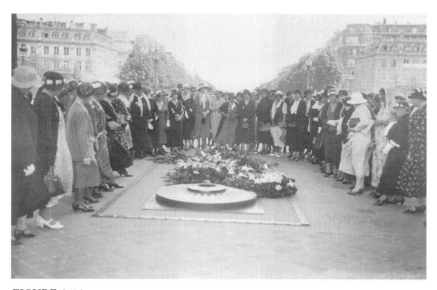

**FIGURE 3-10**
*ICN Members gathered at the Tomb of Unknown Soldiers, Paris, 1933. From AJN Collection.*

lic, she committed herself to lay charity work, visiting the sick at home in some of the poorest Parisian areas. In 1899, she earned a French Red Cross nursing diploma completing her training at La Pitie Hospital. During her career, she initiated many public health programs for the poor in housing, aid for pregnant women and infants, and care for those with tuberculosis. It was she who organized the first professional organization for nurses in France and brought it into the ICN.[60]

In 1931, the treasurer's report was, as usual, the subject of much discussion. Although there was a small credit balance because of voluntary donations by several national associations, the journal was still running a deficit. Once again, Secretary Reimann paid the deficit herself with the usual protestations from the board.

Unemployment for nurses was a worrying global issue. The economic depression of the 1930s affected every aspect of life. A study, presumably conducted by Reimann and authored by her in the ICN's renamed journal, the *International Nursing Review* (INR) in 1933, stated that unemployment was a major problem in "nine out of ten countries" and was "to some extent further aggravated by the unwillingness of the USA to receive the overflow from other nations."[61] Laying the blame on the United States and other industrialized nations, the exchange of nurses was again raised as a possible solution.[62]

## International Exchange Among Nurses

The difficulty nurses found in moving from country to country is illustrated by correspondence during the 1920s and 1930s between the Dutch nursing organization, Nosokomos, and ICN leaders. Most of it was concerned with coordinating exchange opportunities for Dutch nurses to England and the United States.[63] For economic reasons or to increase their international experience, nurses sought positions in the United States or to attend schools of nursing in England or the United States. In 1924, Miss Lloyd Still approved two Dutch nurses who sought to gain some experience in St. Thomas Hospital. Two other nurses were accepted at the Queens Jubilee Institute in 1925.[64] Exchange was difficult for nurses interested in United States experience. Restrictive US immigration laws and employment policies limited foreign nurses' ability to obtain work.[65] Christiane Reimann, who, in 1923, was asked by Nosokomos for help in placing some nurses in the United States, warned the Nosokomos Board that working in the United States would not be easy for foreign nurses. Only a few hospitals would accept them and, if so, only for unpopular chronic cases; usually foreign nurses were not transferred to acute wards.[66] One public health nurse from the Green Cross District Nursing Agency in Utrecht was accepted for half a year as a student at Teachers College in New York.

Usually, successful placements for international work or study experiences were handled on a personal basis. Before a student could be accepted into an American nursing school, her professional standing and the reputation of her training first had to be validated. In the United States, faculty in university schools of nursing, such as Teachers College at Columbia University (New York), many of whom were involved in the ICN, used their network of acquaintances to obtain information on international applicants. When a nurse instructor at the Municipal Hospital of the Hague applied for study at Teachers College, Isabel Stewart first sent a letter to the president of Nosokomos to inquire about the applicant's professional standing.[67] During the first decades of the 20th century, the ICN was still a small community of women from similar backgrounds, who quite easily developed a common understanding of what a good nurse would be. It would not be until after World War II that the increased scale of the ICN, the political complexity of international relationships, the growing diversity of levels of nursing within countries, and the realignments of power among Western countries would change not only the ICN notion of international exchange, but also the question of how to define a good nurse.

## The Third Decade

In 1933, Alicia Lloyd Still took over as president of the ICN. Born in Ceylon in 1869, she grew up in England. As was true of many of her contemporaries, she never had formal schooling and was educated at home by her father. She began her nursing career at a Cottage Hospital in Warminster; then, in 1894, she went to St. Thomas School in London. After finishing at St. Thomas, she went on to become matron of two smaller hospitals. By 1913, she was back at St. Thomas as matron and superintendent of the famous Nightingale school where she remained for 25 years. A forceful personality and self-confessed perfectionist, Lloyd Still was a founding member of the (Royal) College of Nursing in 1916.[68]

At the 1933 Paris-Brussels Congress, ICN Treasurer Musson was finally able to report that, in spite of the worldwide financial crisis, the financial position of the ICN was sound. She seemed to attribute this to the stability of the US dollar, especially because the largest share of the dues came from the Americans. Nevertheless, much discussion continued about problems with member countries' inability to pay dues and monetary exchange rates. Reimann told the congress that she worked and traveled days, nights, and weekends, especially because the assistant editor she hired for the magazine was not satisfactory. She was emphatic at the board of directors meeting that "for ten years she had felt there was too much responsibility on the Secretary." She also complained that it was often

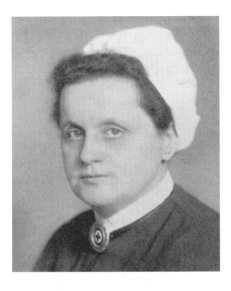

**FIGURE 3-11**
*Anna Schwarzenberg of Austria, Executive Secretary of the ICN 1933 to 1947. From Bridges, A History of the International Council of Nurses, 1967.*

difficult to get help from the president.[69] Between 1925 and 1937, 19 countries became affiliated compared to the 14 who joined between 1899 and 1922. Membership in the ICN membership tripled.

At the 1933 session, the national nurse associations of Austria, Czechoslovakia, Estonia, Hungary, Iceland, and Japan federated with the ICN. The Japanese application to join the ICN gives some sense of how this process worked. According to their 1929 report, the Japanese Nurses Association traced their founding to the Tokyo branch of the Dohokai made up of trained Red Cross nurses. This group advocated for formation of a national union of nurses' organizations and invited some "reliable" ones to join. The founding group included the Tokyo Branch of the Dohokai and alumnae of the training schools of the Medical College of the Imperial University, the Keio University, St. Luke's Hospital, the Jikeikai Hospital, the Saiseikai Hospital, and the Tokyo Private Nurses' Society among others.[70]

## Christiane Reimann Resigns

At the end of the congress, Christiane Reimann announced her intent to resign, prompting the board to reorganize the ICN office. The board decided that future executive secretaries should be assisted by an enlarged staff but should no longer be voting members of the board. In 1934, Princess Anna Schwarzenberg of Austria accepted the position. As was true of Reimann, Schwarzenberg had wide experience of both Europe and America, spoke several languages, and, according to Daisy Bridges, never feared to make her views known.[71]

# Differing Views on Public Health

Concerns about the quality of public health nursing persisted throughout the late 1920s, and in 1931, nursing expert, American Hazel Goff was appointed to the Health Section of the League of Nations for 2 years to advise the League and the ICN on nursing matters. A nurse who was "not a citizen of the United States" donated the money for her salary, which was "on the same scale as that paid to the medical members of the Health Section." Clearly, it was important to the ICN leadership that Goff work on an equal footing with physicians.[72]

American Mary Gardner prepared the report of the ICN Standing Committee on Public Health Nursing for the 1933 Congress. Hazel Goff read the report in Gardner's absence. For 8 years, she said, the committee tried to ascertain the volume and scope of public health nursing in the various countries as well as the type and preparation of those engaged in it. Questionnaires were sent to all regular and corresponding members of the committee, garnering 24 responses, including several from European countries. Eighteen of the 24 responded that satisfactory progress was being made in the development of the field. Mary Gardner was surprised that, especially during the worldwide economic depression, so large a majority was pleased. India was one exception, reporting that there were two few good candidates for public health practice and the country was too poor to fund the enterprise. In many European countries, the question of "who is a trained nurse?" was interpreted differently, making it difficult to compare the qualifications of public health nurses. The countries who said their public health nurses were fully trained often did not include the large number of untrained women actually doing some kind of public health work.

In almost all the countries, women were reported to be doing the work, the majority of which concerned child welfare. Again, the issue of transplanting Western values to non-Western cultures surfaced. For example, one of the national associations that failed to respond to the questionnaire was the Philippine Islands. Almost one third of the 1922 graduates of the public health nursing course from the Philippine General Hospital were men. Alice Fitzgerald, who had started the course with Rockefeller support, believed that men were useful in isolated districts of the country where women could not be sent. Like many of her contemporaries, however, she was generally not supportive of male nurses. She conceded that, given the country's culture and tradition and the safety concerns for women in the bush, men nurses were acceptable in public health nursing.[73]

Just a year later, Hazel Goff's own report on public health nursing in Europe was published.[74] More revealing about a number of issues than the Gardner report, it was ultimately pessimistic about the whole field, although admitting that progress has been made. Goff visited 270 institutions in 10 nonindustrial, rural countries and found that the term *public health nurse* had many meanings. She explained that "ordinarily [public health nurse] refers to a person with more or less hospital experience who either visits in the homes, assists in the consultations, makes social investigations, or attempts to teach the principles of personal and public hygiene" (p. 34). Instead of a graduate nurse, a public health nurse could be parish visitor from a deaconess organization, a health visitor, a social worker, a midwife, feldscher, sanitary inspector, or nutrition worker.

She noted that the functions and objectives of the work were rarely clearly defined. She wrote, "In many organizations there appear to be no specific accomplishments or results sought." In terms of the education of public health nurses, she found that they had very little opportunity to study anything but sick people and that physicians did most of the teaching. Only half of the schools were directed by nurses, and, although most of their graduate nurses were entering the field, only 23 of 50 approved schools actually taught their students about public health.

## The Role of the Rockefeller Foundation

The Rockefeller Foundation was, of course, a major source of funds for many public health programs worldwide—reaching from the United States to China, Europe, and South America during the first 3 decades of the century. Interested in stabilizing society and creating a good environment for capitalist enterprise, Rockefeller executives established public health programs through their International Health Commission. Historians have debated the motives of the foundation, arguing that it sought to improve the health of each country's work force and encourage local economic development to provide the United States with needed raw materials and an adequate market for manufactured goods.[75] According to another view, the foundation was also interested in providing money that would stimulate support from other sources and develop independence in beneficiaries. Edwin Embree, a Rockefeller Foundation decision maker, called these investments "lighthouses."[76] Money would not be given to individuals or to local institutions except those that were established as models for the development of like institutions.[77]

It is clear from reading *The ICN* in the 1920s that the Rockefeller Foundation began its support for schools of nursing all over Europe and the Far East in response to postwar demands for trained public health nurses. Often acting in cooperation with the American Red Cross, which sent its nurses to open the schools, the foundation began its support in the early 1920s to France, Brazil, and schools in Poland and Yugoslavia.[78] In 1929, the foundation reported that maintenance and capital aid in nursing education was being given to schools in Siam, Japan, Lyons (France), Poland, Hungary, Greece and Romania, as well as to American schools. New public health nursing demonstrations were begun in Den-

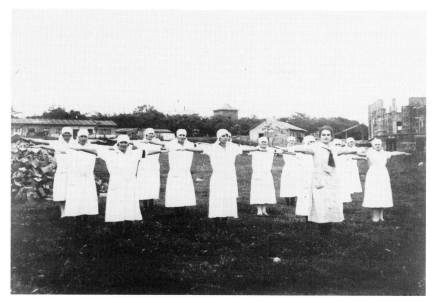

**FIGURE 3-12**
*Nurses at the Belgrade Nurses' Training School, Yugoslavia, 1926. Courtesy of the Rockefeller Archive Center.*

mark and Bulgaria, and the first school of midwifery was given support in Peiping, China in cooperation with the Peiping Union Medical College, also heavily supported by Rockefeller.[79] It is worth noting that many countries joined the ICN a few years after receiving foundation support, for example, France, Poland, and Bulgaria in 1925; Brazil, Philippines, and Yugoslavia in 1929; and Japan, Czechoslovakia, and Hungary in 1933.

Foundation initiatives, by necessity, threaded a way through a fairly complex maze of interested parties seeking postwar roles. For example, the LRCS, as represented by Katherine Olmsted, wanted to enhance its own position concerning public health nursing education. In 1921, she proposed the foundation should make subventions only to the LRCS and not itself undertake any work in nursing.[80] Somewhat in the same vein, leaders of the international course in public health nursing at Bedford College, London, hoped to get some support from Rockefeller as their funds from the LRCS shrank. Edwin Embree, believing the Bedford course to be run by "unimpressive individuals," avoided involvement.[81] Neither the Rockefeller Foundation staff, the American Red Cross leadership, nor, as we have seen, the ICN, supported the LRCS' ambitions, which, at times, extended to oversight of all nursing education organizations in Europe.

In 1921, Rockefeller's International Health Commission was asked for assistance in setting up the first nursing service and school in Brazil. Except for Cuba, there were no schools of nursing in Latin America at this time. The Rockefeller Foundation responded by supporting several American Red Cross nurses in Brazil; by 1923, there were 13 students training in a modern nursing school. Because the demand was especially great for public health nurses, short emergency courses of 10 months were initially given. Eventually, these were discontinued in favor of a new 3-year nursing program.

Rockefeller funded the construction of the Brazilian Anna Nery School as well as a spacious nurses' residence under the direction of American nurse Ethel Parsons.[82] Realizing the importance of establishing a Brazilian nurse as director, Parsons asked public health nurse Rachel Lobo, who had trained in France and received postgraduate education at Teacher's College, Columbia, to succeed her in 1930.[83] This was consistent with American Red Cross practice in many eastern European countries; a nurse leader with citizenship in the country was found as soon as possible.

The foundation was particularly interested in tuberculosis control in France during the war and subsequently cooperated in the development of training schools for nurses and health visitors in Lyons, Strasbourg, Nancy, Lille, and Nantes. According to one author, writing in 1931, the French Central Nursing Bureau was founded in July 1925 *"at the suggestion and with the financial help of the Rockefeller Foundation."* The bureau centralized public health and hospital educational and employment standards.[84]

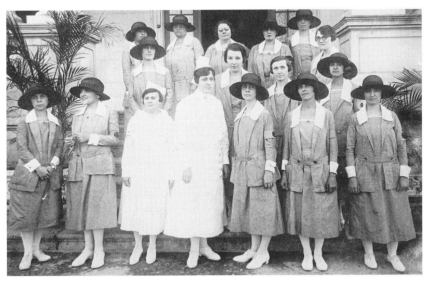

**FIGURE 3-13**
*Public Health Nurses in Rio de Janiero, 1925. From Lynaugh Collection, Bryn Mawr, PA.*

By 1935, the International Health Division of the foundation began to reduce its activities in nursing, only cooperating with governments or educational institutions in the development of schools of nursing where experiments in the education of public health nurses would be made. For example, it gave $250,000 for endowment and $10,000 for equipment to the University School at Brussels, Belgium.[85] Historian Paul Weindling summarized Rockefeller support in eastern Europe between the wars in this way:

> The Rockefeller Foundation supported a public health programme in Eastern Europe which accorded with liberal values in the promoting of public health education, and the development of trained medical administrators, practitioners and scientists. It also wished to enable the successor states to be kept free from German and communist influence . . . . The sustained influence of the International Health Board between 1919 and 1939 enabled every Eastern European Country—apart from the Soviet Union—to establish at least one central Institute for hygiene . . . as well as primary health care programmes designed and financed by the foundation.[86]

## Colonialism—Superior and Subordinate

Contrasting with the Rockefeller Foundation practice of seeking new nursing leadership among citizens of European countries and the Brazil example, a different custom prevailed in British colonies such as India, South Africa, and in the parts of Canada and New Zealand where nonwhite, indigenous populations predominated.[87] In these instances, there is clear evidence of the assumed inferiority of nonwhite groups. Maoris in New Zealand are portrayed in a 1926 article about rural nursing in these racist terms: "he is emerging from race childhood and although highly intelligent he must be treated with consistency and firmness." Special white nurses called "maori nurses" worked in a segregated way with the native people. Nurses for the white population were called "district nurses."[88] In Australia, an article on conditions for nurses stated that nurses were "eminently practical" and would do anything because "there are no inferior races to do the so-called menial work."[89]

In India, a photograph taken at the 1929 Annual Conference of Trained Nurses tells us much about the integration of native nurses in the British colony. There are 6 Indian nurses on the margins of a picture of 40 white nurses.[90] An earlier article, written by Miss Bonser, the British superintendent of nursing at a Dehli Hospital, tells us about the "charity model" of development of nursing services in the colonies, as well as about the stigma around the work of nursing for contemporary Indians.

Bonser pointed out that hospitals all over the country were started by government aid or by medical missions. European and American women worked in India for years, and private nursing was almost entirely in their hands because "purdah customs . . . make it almost indecent for an unmarried Indian girl to visit patients in their own homes unattended."[91] Thus, according to another source, medical missionaries actively encouraged Christian women (and men) to train as nurses because "Hindu parents were held back by the deep seated inhibitions of caste from allowing their daughters to take up [nursing], while Muslim girls were prohibited under the purdah system from showing themselves in public."[92] At the time of World War II, some 90% of Indian nurses came from the small Christian community and 80% of all Indian nurses had been trained in mission hospitals.[93]

In 1930, Ethel Watts wrote that many of the large hospitals in India were run by European or American nurses, but that many (smaller) hospitals were headed by Indians. Nevertheless, Lady Symon, the wife of Sir Henry Symon, director general of the Indian Medical Service, served as the president of the Trained Nurses Association of India. Watts concluded, a little defensively, that "it remains for the Indian nurse to rise up and possess the land. Where there are Indian nurses ready to take responsible positions they have ample opportunities."[94]

Because Great Britain controlled the largest Western colonial empire for over 75 years, it is not surprising that much discussion centers on British practices abroad. In the case of India, for example, it is clear that both direct and indirect imperial systems were used by British colonizers. How did these two systems work? Direct imperialism meant that British interests were promoted and protected by abolishing indigenous administrative institutions and social practices in favor of new ruling institutions and bureaucracies. In this model, a small number of Western salaried agents were hired at the higher levels helped by selected indigenous men at the lower echelons. By contrast, in colonies administered by indirect imperialism, traditional political institutions and social practices were maintained, subject to treaties or agreements with the traditional rulers and administered by resident agents whose aim was to accomplish colonial objectives through the facade of indigenous leadership.[95]

Sounding an attitude that one historian has called "maternal imperialism," Bonser wrote that "one cannot write of Nursing in India without reference to the great help which has always been given by the wives of Viceroys and Governors to further this work . . . all monuments to those ladies who recognized the great need for an efficient nursing service in this country."[96] Maternal imperialism may fairly characterize many of the nurses and Christian missionaries who, while sympathetic to Indians, generally subscribed to the notion of superiority of their own culture and political systems. These reform-minded women were frequently referred to as mothers, or saw themselves as mothering India and Indians.[97]

Few other mission fields attracted such high proportions of women missionary doctors and nurses as India. It was considered vitally important that women medical and nursing missionaries reach into the *zenana*, the exclusively female quarters within Indian households where both Muslim and Hindu women were secluded. No male medical attendant was permitted here for attendance at childbirth. This meant that indigenous midwives (called *dais*) had been the preferred attendants. They were often characterized by Europeans as dangerous because they were said to be untrained, and thus ignorant of asepsis and control of hemorrhage.[98]

In the early 1930s, several articles propounding the necessity to Christianize "natives" in South Africa appeared in the ICN journal. In one, the Bantus of Africa were portrayed as having a "primitive" mentality and believing in witchcraft. The author, anthropologist Johanne Larsen, wrote, "We Europeans, who reflect and reason, experience an irresistible need to understand everything, to be logical. The Bantu does not reason, knows nothing of logic, does not examine things. He can therefore believe that even the smallest malady, if it be a cold or toothache, is caused by witchcraft." Larsen further recommended that "we must help them to emerge from the daily terror and fear of the unknown occult power around them, and to ground their faith on the true foundations of Christianity, which casts out fear."[99]

In a second piece, physician E. D. Earthy exhaustively describes the extent of infant mortality among natives in South Africa, concluding that "a great forward movement should be made . . . in a long, patient and prolonged effort in Christian Education and against superstition . . . and in encouraging and supporting the work of Christian missions, which have always been the pioneers of both medical and moral advance among the different tribal groups." Earthy also called for more native hospitals, doctors, and nurses. Although the economic conditions of the natives were cited as the first reason for the mortality, material amelioration was not recommended.[100]

Despite calls for more native practitioners in South Africa, all members of the South African Trained Nurses Association were "white people" in 1922 when the association was voted into full membership by the ICN.[101] Native (presumably black or "colored" indigenous women) nurses were trained in a few mission hospitals or at the Non European Hospital in Johannesburg. According to Miss B. G. Alexander, general secretary of the South African Trained Nurses Association, native women were trained as early as 1903 at the Lovedal Mission, although they were not eligible for state registration. In 1927, she reported that "the numbers are not large, but so far ten of its graduates are now state-registered." She went on to say that "the hospital has a European [white] Matron and Sister, under whose directions the nursing is done by sixteen native student nurses."[102]

Another article in the same issue describing the native nurse of South Africa ("her problems and her future") noted there were "probably not more than half a dozen" training schools for black women in all South

Africa. The "native" population was 5.5 million at this time. Christiane Reimann's editor's note points out that the "natives" outnumbered whites "by about three to one." It is clear from these sources how marginalized and segregated black women were and how few nurses were trained from their population.

Given these examples, it seems reasonable to ask how ICN leaders thought about the differences that existed between them and women living in some of the so-called non-Western countries. Historian Mervat Hatem concludes her study of how European and non-European women of the time saw each other this way:

> By accepting the contention that they were superior to women from other cultures, European women's attention was diverted from the fact that they continued to be subordinate to European and other men with whom they came into contact.[103]

In many, if not all, colonized countries, there was an explicit assumption that the white race was superior; or, as historian Vron Ware put it, the problem of difference was really the problem of privilege, that is, "in a society habituated to dominant ideologies of white supremacy it is often easier for people who fall in the category 'white' to see themselves as merely 'normal' and therefore without a racialized identity." Therefore, ideas about what constituted white femininity in the 1920s and 1930s were constructed in relation to those about black femininity and vice versa.[104]

It is plain that complex interactions between ideologies of gender, race, and class became ever more problematic in the 1920s and 1930s during unprecedented expansion in the organization. Indeed, it is difficult to untangle these layers of beliefs. Of course, some ICN leaders continued to assert, as did Ethel Gordon Fenwick at the 1925 ICN Congress, that *there is no nationality in nursing* (her emphasis).

In actual practice, however, attitudes toward race and class were revealed in the ways that indigenous people were sometimes marginalized or ignored as nurses in their own countries. The charity model of nursing development in some countries, the often unspoken criteria for deciding on acceptable member countries, the question of who should represent a country at the ICN, the assumed superiority of Western women and their nursing systems, and the complicity with colonial and imperial sensibilities, all acted to verify the reality of Lavinia Dock's "lurking shades of difference."

## Comradeship

So, it seems the imagined community of the ICN was broadening but was still inherently limited by Dock's "lurking shades" and by the rules governing who could, or could not, join. Still, some things were different now. The only partially realized, but great potential of this imagined community and the support of a worldwide organization were demonstrated in 1929, when a nurse in the Philippines was accused and convicted of "homicide through reckless imprudence." Her national association defended her and lobbied on her behalf to the ICN and to government officials until she was pardoned. Her crime had been to give a surgeon the drug that he had ordered to be injected. The drug was harmful and killed the patient. (The physician was exonerated.) An ICN summary of the case concluded,

> One of the finest results of the Somera Case is the strengthening of professional consciousness in our group. The humblest nurse in the farthest place in the Philippine Islands is no longer an isolated, forlorn worker, but a part of a great organism that not only suffers when she suffers and rejoices when she is made glad, but is ready with advice and help—the International Council of Nurses.[105]

## ENDNOTES

1. Christiane Reimann was appointed Honorary Secretary, the post held by Lavinia Dock. In 1925, when the ICN reorganized, her full-time involvement was recognized by the title Executive Secretary, a post she held until 1934.

2. For more details on Sophie Mannerheim, see the International Council of Nurses' Swedish translation of Berta Edelfelt's *En Levnadstecking*, 1929, Columbia University Teachers College Archives, Adelaide Nutting Collection, AN 1054, New York, New York, USA. See also Tyyni Tuulio, *Sophie Mannerheim* (Helsinki: Foundation of Nursing Education, 1963) translated to English by Brad Absetz, and "Sophie Mannerheim, Abstracts From a Memoir," *The Canadian Nurse*, 27 (October 1931): 10–12. We are very grateful to Dr. Marianne Tallberg of Helsingfors, Finland, who shared her research and expertise on Sophie Mannerheim and her era.

3. Breay and Fenwick, 142.

4. Bridges, 66–67.

5. The Round Table on Professional Ethics was transcribed in *The ICN*, 1 (January 1926): 23–28. ICNA.

6. Ibid., 26. Mlle. Chaptal would become ICN president in 1929.

7. Mary Louise Roberts, "'This Civilization No Longer Has Sexes': *La Garconne* and Cultural Crisis in France After World War One," *Gender and History*, 4, (Spring 1992): 64.

8. Sandra Gwyn, *Tapestry of War. A Private View of Canadians in the Great War* (Toronto: Harper Collins Publishers, 1992), xvii.

9. E. H. Carr, *The Twenty Years' Crisis, 1919–1939*, 2nd ed. (London: Macmillan and Co. Ltd, 1946), 224.

10. Ibid., see 226–228. See also E. J. Hobsbawm, *Nations and Nationalism Since 1780. Programme, Myth, Reality* (Cambridge: Cambridge University Press, 1990) as well as Raymond Aron, *The Century of Total War* (Boston: The Beacon Press, 1955).

11. Martin Kitchen, *Europe Between the Wars. A Political History* (Harlow: Longman, 1988), 20. Although none of the Allies doubted Germany's guilt in causing and prolonging losses in the war, Germans never accepted the guilt, nor, as Kitchen explains, that they had lost the war.

12. *The ICN*, Bulletin 1 (January 1924): 28.
13. Quotations from a letter from Agnes Karll, *The ICN*, Bulletin 2 (April 1924): 40. ICNA.
14. Alexandra Romanoff, "Russian Nurses and Nursing," *The ICN*, 1 (April 1926): 119. ICNA.
15. Alexandra Romanoff, "Russian Nurses and Nursing," *The ICN*, 1 (January 1926): 32–33. ICNA.
16. Romanoff, (April 1926): 122.
17. Ibid., 117–123, especially 120 and note on page 121.
18. Anna J. Haines, *Health Work in Soviet Russia* (New York: Vanguard Press, 1928).
19. Bridges, 54.
20. Christiane Reimann, "The Past Is Inspiring," *International Nursing Review*, 6, (July 1959): 7.
21. Fenwick was irritated that a special meeting was called and declined to attend, citing the expense and irregularity of the special meeting. Ethel G. Fenwick to Christiane Reimann, 5 May 1923, Mannerheim Correspondence (courtesy of M. Tallberg).
22. See Summers, *Angels and Citizens*, Chapter 9, for the VADs and how they were deployed. See Vera Brittain, *Testament of Youth* (Great Britain: Victor Gollancz Ltd., 1933) [original] for a first-hand account of a VAD and the hostility she encountered from trained nurses.
23. See Bridget Towers and John Hutchinson in Paul Weindling, Ed., *International Health Organizations During the Inter-War Period* (Cambridge: Cambridge University Press, 1995). See also John F. Hutchinson, *Champions of Charity* (Boulder, CO: Westview Press, 1996).
24. Lavinia Dock, "Foreign Department: The Next International," *American Journal of Nursing*, 19 (November 1919): 870.
25. Lavinia Dock, "Foreign Department: International Public Health Department," *American Journal of Nursing*, 21 (May 1921): 316.
26. Elizabeth Fox, "The Work of the Nursing Advisory Board of the League of Red Cross Societies," *The ICN*, Bulletin 3 (July 1924): 36–41, ICNA; Bridges, 59–60, and Mannerheim Correspondence (courtesy of M. Tallberg).
27. Mary S. Gardner, "Changing Emphasis in Public Health Nursing," *The ICN*, 1 (January 1926): 42.
28. For events in the period, see Anne Marie Rafferty, "Internationalizing Nursing Education During the Interwar Period," Weindling, *International Health Organizations*, 266–282.
29. Christiane Reimann, "Two International Courses for Nurses, Bedford College, University of London, England," *The ICN*, Bulletin 4 (October 1924): 34–35, ICNA. For information on scholarships provided by the Rockefeller Foundation, see "Miscellaneous," Ibid., 51. See also the report on fellowships in nursing awarded for training in "Current Events—The Rockefeller Foundation Annual Report, 1929," *International Nursing Review*, V, (November 1930), np.
30. See minutes of the Nursing Advisory Board of the LRCS, April 23–29, 1924, ICNA. See also Mannerheim Correspondence (courtesy of M. Tallberg).
31. Ibid.
32. Nutting letter to Mannerheim, 28 May 1923, Mannerheim Correspondence (courtesy of M. Tallberg). A native of Wisconsin in the United States, Olmsted had served as a Red Cross nurse in Romania during World War I, surviving a harrowing escape from the Germans; a graduate of Johns Hopkins Training School for Nurses she also

worked as an executive secretary of the National Organization of Public Health Nurses' Western office before moving on in 1921 to the LRCS. Signe S. Cooper, "Katherine M. Olmsted," Vern Bullough, et al, Eds. *American Nursing: A Biographical Dictionary* (New York and London: Garland Publishing Co., 1988), 247–248.

33. Letters 6 January 1927 and her reply 18 January 1927, Mannerheim Correspondence (courtesy of M. Tallberg). Mannerheim would never have the opportunity to accept the position. Developing a serious illness, she died in March 1928.

34. Ethel G. Fenwick to Christiane Reimann, 23 May 1923, Mannerheim Correspondence (courtesy of M. Tallberg).

35. See Breay, 143–147 for Fenwick's letter to the council. The full story is told in detail elsewhere. See especially Susan McGann, *The Battle of the Nurses* (London: Scutari Press, 1992). Also, see Rafferty, *The Politics of Nursing Knowledge*. Conflicts over control of British nursing remained an international issue during the entire interwar period.

36. Sophie Mannerheim wrote to Adelaide Nutting in September 1924 reporting that she, "begged [Mrs. Fenwick] to find some way out of this distressing situation" because the majority of British nurses, who were represented by the College of Nursing, could not, under the circumstances, be members of ICN. She also confessed to Nutting that she (Mannerheim) told Mrs. Fenwick that she "could not remain with her" to hear Mrs. Fenwick's abuse of nurses from Mannerheim's alma mater, St. Thomas Hospital in London. Sophie Mannerheim to Adelaide Nutting, 17 September 1924, Mannerheim Correspondence (courtesy of M. Tallberg).

37. Sophie Mannerheim to Clara Noyes, 28 April 1925, Mannerheim Correspondence (courtesy of M. Tallberg).

38. Ibid., 31.

39. Bridges, 61.

40. Minutes, Board of Directors of International Council of Nurses, Geneva, 1927, p. 17, ICNA.

41. Kaiyi Chen, "Missionaries and the Early Development of Nursing in China," *Nursing History Review*, 4 (1996): 129–149. Dr. Chen's use of both Chinese and Western sources make his work on this period unique.

42. Ibid., 129.

43. Chen, "Missionaries": 135.

44. Nina Gage and Ruth Ingram, "Nursing Education in Universities in China," *The ICN*, 2 (1927): 83–95. This report on Chinese nursing reflects existing imperialist relationships.

45. Ibid.

46. *The ICN*, 1 (1926): 298–299. For Rockefeller, see E. Richard Brown, *Rockefeller Medicine Men, Medicine and Capitalism in America* (Berkeley: University of California Press, 1979), 116. See also Kaiyi Chen, "Quality Versus Quantity: The Rockefeller Foundation and Nurses' Training in China," *The Journal of American-East Asian Relations*, 5 (Spring 1996): 77–104.

47. *The ICN*, 2 (1927): 83–95. For a detailed discussion of the life and times of the Peking Union Medical College and its nursing program, see Kaiyi Chen, "Quality Versus Quantity."

48. *The ICN*, Bulletin 4 (October 1924): 42–44.

49. Chen, "Missionaries": 140.

50. *The ICN*, Bulletin 5 (Winter 1925): 7–8.

51. *The ICN*, 2 (1927): 61. *The ICN*, Bulletin 4 (October 1924): 42–44. ICNA.

52. *American Journal of Nursing,* 22 (November 1922): 918–920.

53. Quoted in Chen, "Missionaries": 141.

54. For an analysis of these issues, see Susan Reverby, "A Legitimate Relationship: Nursing, Hospitals, and Science in the Twentieth Century," in Diana Long and Janet Golden, Eds. *The American General Hospital* (Ithaca: Cornell University Press, 1989), 135–156. See also Isabel Maitland Stewart, *The Education of Nurses—Historical Foundations and Modern Trends* (New York and London: Garland Publishing, 1984). [Originally, Macmillan, 1950.]

55. Its first comprehensive document on nursing education was published by ICN in 1930. See "Report of the Committee on Education of the International Council of Nurses," Annex to the Minutes of the Meeting of the Grand Council, Paris, 1933, ICNA. The committee chair was an American, Isabel Stewart. This document was widely circulated and reprinted and was also used by the League of Red Cross Societies as a guide in developing nursing education.

56. In 1915, Goodrich proclaimed at the San Francisco ICN meeting, "We shall not rest until institutions of higher learning as well as institutions for the sick, have opened their doors for our members." Rebecca Strong, who made her career at the Glasgow Royal Infirmary, strove to base nursing education in the university and was credited by Goodrich for her early achievements. See McGann, *The Battle of the Nurses,* 124 and passim.

57. Isabel Stewart, "Report of the Committee, 1933," ICNA.

58. Minutes, Grand Council of the International Council of Nurses, Montreal, 1929, ICNA.

59. Bridges, 86.

60. For more on the history of nursing in France, see Y. Knibiehler, *Cornettes et Blouses Blanches—Les Infirmeries dans la Societe Francaise* [Caps or White Blouses—Nursing in French Society, 1880–1980] (France: Hachette, 1984); Geertje Boschma, "Review of Selected Histories."

61. Editorial, "The Recruiting of Nursing Staff," *International Nursing Review,* VII (1933): 1–11.

62. Henny Tscherning had encouraged such exchanges during her tenure as ICN president.

63. Boxes 128, 133, 134, 148–151, Nosokomos Archives, Municipal Archives Amsterdam.

64. Box 133, Nosokomos Archives.

65. Letter of the American Consulate, 23-6-1923, Box 128, Nosokomos Archives.

66. Correspondence With ICN, 1923, Box 148, Nosokomos Archives.

67. Letter of Isabel Stewart to Miss Verwey, 16 February 1928, Box 128, Nosokomos Archives.

68. Lucy Seymer, *Dame Alicia Lloyd Still, 1869–1944—A Memoir* (London: The Nightingale Fellowship, St. Thomas Hospital, 1953).

69. International Council of Nurses, Board of Directors Minutes, Paris, July 1933, p. 26. ICNA. See also "Report of Special Committee Appointed by the Board to Consider Possible Reorganization of the Headquarters Office, 1933," in which much tighter controls on the secretary and the office were recommended.

70. The Japan Nurses Association, Report, Montreal, Canada, 1929. p. 5, ICNA.

71. Bridges, 92–95.

72. "A Nursing Expert Appointed," *International Nursing Review,* VI (September 1931): 483.

73. See Barbara Brush, "Unexpected Consequences: The Rockefeller Agenda for American/Philippine Nursing Relations," *Western Journal of Nursing Research*, 17(5): 540–555.

74. Hazel Goff, "Report of a Study of Public Health Nursing in Europe," *International Nursing Review*, IX (1934): 31–45.

75. E. Richard Brown, *Rockefeller Medicine Men. Medicine and Capitalism in America* (Berkeley: University of California Press, 1979), 116.

76. Rafferty, "Internationalizing Nursing Education," 272.

77. Sarah Abrams, "Brilliance and Bureaucracy. Nursing and Changes in the Rockefeller Foundation, 1915–1930," *Nursing History Review*, 1 (1993): 123. See p. 119. Rockefeller used this model in the United States; between 1918 and 1930, they contributed $2.3 million to nursing education and practice.

78. "Miscellaneous," *The ICN*, Bulletin 5 (Winter 1925): 62. *The ICN*, under the editorship of Reimann until 1933, was always careful to report Rockefeller news, although the October 1924 issue reported that "the R.F. prefers as little as possible mentioned about what they are doing" (p. 51).

79. *International Nursing Review*, V (November 1930): 613.

80. Rafferty, "Internationalizing Nursing Education," 274.

81. Ibid., 275.

82. Ethel Parsons, "Modern Nursing in Brazil," *The ICN*, 2, (1927): 292–298.

83. "Rachel Haddock Lobo" (Obituary), *International Nursing Review*, IX (1934): 4–5. Unfortunately, Lobo died in 1933 at the age of 42, only 3 years after taking over in 1930. She founded the first professional nursing journal in Brazil.

84. Mlle. J. Delagrange, "Le Bureau Central des Infirmieres Aupres de la Sante Publique de L'Etat Francais," *International Nursing Review*, VI (January 1931): 60–63.

85. "Here and There with the Rockefeller Foundation," *International Nursing Review*, XI (1937): 270–274.

86. Paul Weindling, "Public Health and Political Stabilization: The Rockefeller Foundation in Central and Eastern Europe Between the Two World Wars," *Minerva*, 31 (Autumn 1993): 265–266.

87. There have never been many trained aboriginal nurses in Canada—until the 1950s, virtually none. For a fascinating insight into 18th and 19th century European attitudes to northern Inuit people in Canada, see Walter Vanast, "'Ignorant of Any Rational Method: European Assessments of Indigenous Healing Practices in the North American Arctic," *Canadian Bulletin of Medical History*, 9 (1992), 57–69.

88. A. Bagley, "Back Block Nursing in New Zealand," *The ICN*, 1 (July 1926): 169. In contrast to this attitude, a more integrated service model appeared in the early 1930s, with the "European" (ie, white) district nurse (in at least one instance) working closely with the Maoris to adapt their culture to preventive health care practices. See Helen Campbell, *Mary Lambie—A Biography* (Wellington, New Zealand: Nursing Education and Research Foundation, 1976). Lambie was a public health nurse and leader in New Zealand nursing as well as holding several key elected positions in the ICN in the 1940s and 1950s.

89. J. Bell, "Nursing Conditions and Problems in Australia," *The ICN*, 1 (April 1926): 124.

90. The photograph is reproduced in the May 1930 issue of the *International Nursing Review*.

91. Miss Bonser, "Short Summary of Nursing Work in India During Recent Years," *The ICN*, Bulletin 6 (Spring 1925): 36–37. In a footnote to Miss Bonser's article, Reimann

wrote that in the Bombay section of India, Hindu, Christian and Parsee Indian women worked among their communities as private-duty nurses and were well respected. Nursing work was not seen this way in most parts of India, however.

92. Alice Wilkinson, *A Brief History of Nursing in India and Pakistan* (NP: The Trained Nurses' Association of India, 1958), 31. Alice Wilkinson was a white British nurse who had been the nursing superintendent of a mission hospital in Delhi from 1908 to 1938. Her picture appears in the book. Her association with Indian nursing "for more than forty years" was apparently at least part of the reason she was asked to write the history, according to the Foreword by Rajkumari A. Kaur.

93. Quoted on p. 11 in Rosemary Fitzgerald, "Rescue and Redemption: The Rise of Female Medical Missions in Colonial India in the Late 19th and Early 20th Centuries." Paper presented to the conference, Nursing, Women's History and the Politics of Welfare, University of Nottingham, England, July 1993.

94. Ethel Watts, "The Training of Nurses in India: Its Problems and Prospects," *International Nursing Review*, V (May 1930): 228–235.

95. Nupur Chaudhuri and Margaret Strobel, Eds. *Western Women and Imperialism—Complicity and Resistance* (Bloomington, IN: Indiana University Press, 1992), "Introduction," 5.

96. Bonser, "Short Summary of Nursing Work in India": 36–37.

97. For a discussion of how this worked, see Barbara Ramusack, "Cultural Missionaries, Maternal Imperialists, Feminist Allies. British Women Activists in India, 1865–1945," in Chaudhuri and Strobel, Eds. *Western Women and Imperialism*, pp. 119–136. See also Dea Birkett, "The White Woman's Burden in the White Man's Grave: The Introduction of British Nurses in Colonial West Africa," pp. 177–188.

98. For zenanas, see Fitzgerald; for a description of the "dais" and how the official history of Indian nursing viewed them, see Wilkinson, 57–64.

99. Johanne Larsen, "The Bantu Conception of Illness," *International Nursing Review*, V (November 1930): 552–557.

100. E. D. Earthy, "Stillbirth and Infantile Mortality in South Africa from the Social and Economic Point of View," *International Nursing Review*, 6 (July 1931): 343–363.

101. International Council of Nurses, Council Meeting, New Business, Copenhagen, Denmark, May 1922, p. 47. ICNA.

102. "Current Events," *The ICN*, 2 (July 1927): 244. See also Michael Gelfand, *Christian Doctor and Nurse* (Atholi, Sandton, SA: Privately published, 1984).

103. Mervat Hatem, "Through Each Other's Eyes: The Impact on the Colonial Encounter of the Images of Egyptian, Levantine-Egyptian, and European Women, 1862–1920," in Chaudhuri and Strobel, p. 56.

104. Vron Ware, "Moments of Danger: Race, Gender and Memories of Empire," *History and Theory*, 31 (1992): 118–119.

105. Elizabeth Grennan, "The Somera Case," *International Nursing Review*, V (July 1930): 325–333.

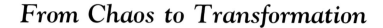

# From Chaos to Transformation

*JOAN E. LYNAUGH*

*I*n no way could the leadership and staff of the International Council of Nurses (ICN), in the years immediately preceding World War II, comprehend what the future held for them. World War II and its dislocations would prove to be the defining event for the organization and its members. The ICN, as was true of all nursing, was about to be caught up and ultimately transformed by a time of worldwide destruction, personal tragedy, political realignment, and economic upheaval. Influence over the inner workings of the ICN shifted away from Europe and toward the United States and Canada during and after the war. Then, during the 1950s, the ICN's Anglo-Eurocentric character underwent a fundamental change as new members were introduced from Africa, Asia, and South America. With this expansion, the ICN finally began to actually implement its new, more global agenda.

Some ICN leaders hoped and worked for the ICN to become a stronger participant in postwar internationalism, and gradually it did. However, the political barriers of the East–West Cold War and continuing racial, religious, and gender issues tempered, complicated, and sometimes delayed implementing broader ICN goals even after the wartime chaos faded away. In spite of these obstacles, the longstanding objectives of the ICN—internationalism, professionalism, and standardization of nursing—would come ever closer to reality during the 25 years after 1945.

## Struggling to Keep the ICN Alive

In 1937, however, ICN officers were still caught up in the familiar dilemmas caused by financial constraint, limited staff, and overly ambitious agendas. The internal personnel problems of the struggling organization were reflected in President Alicia Lloyd Still's 1937 final report to the council, as she told of the chaos she found in 1933 when she took office. Still fresh in her mind were all the problems associated with the transfer of office management from Christiane Reimann to Princess Anna Schwarzenberg.[1] Lloyd Still complained that the ICN office in Geneva was in great disorganization and further charged that the departing Reimann took with her unspecified ICN documents pertaining to hiring staff and other confidential papers. Citing lack of funds, Lloyd Still explained that she had to "suspend further publications of the *International Nursing Review*" in 1934.

Continuing her report on a more positive note, Lloyd Still characterized the years between 1935 and 1937 as years of "reconstruction" for the ICN. Indeed, by 1936, she again found it possible to publish the ICN journal. The 1937 ICN move back to London was planned, in part, to take advantage of a better rate of exchange, but also, as Schwarzenberg remarked, because some ICN decision makers saw London as the "centre of the nursing world."[2] This view contrasted with the opinion of the Rockefeller Foundation staff and probably irritated American nurse leaders. Money continued to be a severe problem, but the tone of the 1937 London meeting conveyed the sense that the board believed the ICN was getting back on its feet after several trying years.

A united Australian nursing association, an internationally minded Switzerland, and Rumania all joined the ICN in 1937, bringing the total number of national nurse association members to 32.[3] Daisy Bridges recalled the congress as lively, with a conventionlike atmosphere and much pomp. Americans Mary Beard and Elizabeth Crowell, Rockefeller Foundation staffers in the United States and Europe, respectively, were given honorary membership at the 1937 ICN Congress. Their citation read, "through the interest and far reaching vision of these nurses, individual countries affiliated with the ICN have profited immeasurably and have been enabled to advance materially their nursing services and their nursing education, to the advantage of social welfare work in the whole world."[4] The Beard and Crowell honors also symbolized continued interest and

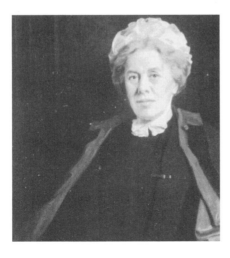

**FIGURE 4-1**
*Alicia Lloyd Still, ICN President 1933 to 1937. From Bridges, A History of the International Council of Nurses, 1967.*

commitment among the ICN leadership to the public health ideal. Rockefeller Foundation links with nursing and public health dated from its post World War I efforts in France. In retrospect, it looks as though the foundation's nursing agenda was largely predicated to serve its goals for medicine and disease control. The ICN leadership, however, preferred to emphasize the influence and importance for nursing in Europe of the Foundation-commissioned nursing surveys by American Annie Goodrich, Britain's Daisy Bridges and later Canadian Kathleen Russell.

Amidst the pomp and good feelings, however, striking differences in interpreting the unstable political world situation permeated the 1937 Board Meeting and Grand Council. An excerpt illustrates the barely papered-over dissent among the members. In the council, the Canadian Nurses Association (CNA) recommended that "the ICN stress to the women of the world their united effort to sponsor and support measures for the promotion of world peace and control of armaments."[5] Those arguing against the Canadian recommendation raised the point that peace and armament control were political questions which ICN should avoid. Miss Helen Dey of Great Britain thought the ICN should not have "any-

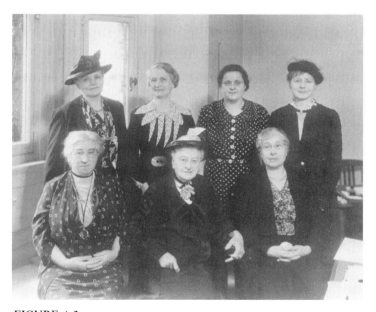

**FIGURE 4-2**

*ICN group in London, 1937. Seated: Ellen Musson, Ethel Gordon Fenwick, Effie Taylor. Standing: Jeanne de Joannis (France), Bella Alexander (South Africa), Anna Schwarzenberg, and Bertha Hegelstad (Norway). From Bridges, A History of the International Council of Nurses, 1967.*

thing to do with control of armaments," and, in Fenwick's view, "control of armaments could not really be considered without a political bias."[6] In her support of military preparedness, Fenwick remained perfectly consistent with her pre-World War I position. Recognizing the wide gap in perceptions of the world situation among council members, and seeing such differing beliefs about the function of the ICN, Grace Fairley of Canada withdrew the CNA recommendation.

This debate and its outcome were consistent with the prewar ICN's aversion to political controversy and the leadership's reluctance to engage each other on any issues outside of nursing. Perhaps uneasiness about the future and the tensions created by opposing views helped inspire Lloyd Still's selection of the watchword "loyalty" for the next 4 years. She exhorted her listeners to strive for "loyalty to your country, loyalty to your Vocation, loyalty to your Womanhood."[7] Lloyd Still reminded her nurse audience of their dual roles as representatives of their countries and worldwide caretakers of the sick. As was true for the generation before them, these nurse-citizens were face to face with the dilemma imposed by loyalty to their own countries in a time of intense nationalism versus the competing ideal of the universalist obligations of professionalism.

The 1937 London Congress elected Euphemia J. (Effie) Taylor of Yale University as the new president, making her actually the third ICN president from the United States. Annie Goodrich preceded her in 1912. Nina Gage, who was living in China when elected ICN president, was a US citizen. Taylor was destined to remain president for 10 years, throughout the war, until the Ninth Congress in 1947.

Taylor was born in Hamilton, Ontario, Canada in 1874. She was educated in Canada; in 1908, she graduated from the nursing program at Johns Hopkins Hospital School of Nursing in Baltimore, Maryland, USA. Later, she earned a baccalaureate at Teachers College, Columbia University in New York City. She was well known in psychiatric nursing circles, but made her career in leadership posts in nursing education after assuming the deanship at Yale University School of Nursing in 1934. Before accepting the post at the ICN, she had served as president of the National League of Nursing Education (NLNE) during the early 1930s.

Congress participant, postwar ICN executive secretary, and ICN historian Daisy Bridges chose, in her 1967 history, to highlight the 1937 Congress with this quote from a closing speaker, which in the light of subsequent events, has poignant overtones: "We are carrying home new ideas for development, but these are not of first importance. It is friendship with one another that makes and keeps the ICN a living thing."[8] The loyalties and friendships of the leaders and members of the ICN would be challenged and interrupted almost immediately, for, even as the congress met, nursing, as they understood it, was being pulled apart.

In Germany, under national socialism, nurses were, at first, segregated into separate organizations; there was one for Roman Catholics, for the

Protestant sisterhoods, for Red Cross nurses, and one for the new National-ist-Socialist Sisterhood, who mostly worked in public health. As to the latter, "Their main task is to educate the public to understand that each individual, as a member of the state, has the duty of keeping himself and his family in good health."[9] A fifth organization, the National Union of Independent Sisters and Nurses, was set up by the government to absorb all other nurses. The 1937 ICN Council heard this report of extensive nursing change in Germany, but the records reveal no comment or criti-cism from the listeners.

For its next step, the Third Reich government decreed in 1938 that all nurses must join some group or eventually forfeit their right to practice. The National Socialist Welfare Organization set up public nursing centers in distant parts of Germany; the improved economy employed more nurses, which eased the devastating nurse unemployment of the early 1930s. His-torian Hilda Steppe quotes the oath taken by Nazi community nurses. "I solemnly swear that I will be steadfastly faithful and obedient to Adolf Hitler, my Fuhrer. I promise to fulfill my duties, wherever I may be desig-nated to work, faithfully and conscientiously as a national-socialist nurse in service to the national community, so help me God."[10]

Then, in July 1939, the ICN Board heard Frau Oberin Blunck sorrow-fully report the dissolution of the professional Nurses' Association of Ger-many of which she was president in favor of the Reich's Union of German Nurses and Nursing Assistants. "I ask you to believe that the German nurses are still interested, as they have always been, in maintaining and furthering this cooperation," she said. Invoking the memory of Agnes Karll, she pleaded for some way to continue connections with the ICN.[11] The ICN Board could only stand by and witness the crumbling and corrup-tion of professional independence and values so painstakingly erected over nearly 4 decades in Germany—one of ICN's three founding nations.

Taylor's presidential message to the board in July 1939 struck an al-most wistful note. Some of her language, seemingly, denied the reality around her. "From China and Japan [already at war with each other for some 3 years] letters have come which make us proud of the work that, under danger and privation, has been accomplished by the nurses in both these lands . . . at no time has there been indication or expression of enmity or bitterness on the part of nurses—only sorrowful thought for those who suffer and anxiety that enough may not be accomplished to meet their needs." And later in her message, she pled, " . . . as members of thirty and more affiliated countries, may we demonstrate to our individual nations that insignificant problems have no place in marring our relation-ships, and that as human beings we will have differences of opinion on minor issues, but we are harmonious on the objectives which count and for which our organization stands."[12]

At this meeting, the ICN learned of the dissolution of the Austrian Nurses Association by the German Third Reich after Hitler's establishment of the National Socialist government of Austria—another loss to the ICN that hardly seems "insignificant." Executive Secretary Anna Schwarzenberg, now an Austrian without a national association, quickly had to ally herself with the Swiss Nurses Association so she could remain in the ICN.

Schwarzenberg's own report to the board is more revealing of the turmoil generated by war in Europe. She listed a chronicle of changes: an ICN staff member gave up her job and returned to Germany; Calista Banwarth, an American enrolled in the International course at Bedford College in London, pressed into service to cope with the backlog of work; a Jewish refugee forced to flee from Germany and given work on the ICN staff; and the office's heavy involvement in finding nursing work for other nurse refugees from Germany and other parts of Europe.

As soon as the council meeting was over, Schwarzenberg planned to go to South Africa and India to visit the national nurse associations there. She did leave in early August 1939 and was aboard ship in September when war broke out; she abandoned the trip and returned to London. Recognizing the implications of her personal situation as a member of a titled Austrian family, she requested a leave of absence, briefly visited her home in Austria, and then went to Spain. Later, with Taylor's help, she made her way to the United States.

ICN Treasurer Ellen Musson saw and understood the serious implications of the world situation. In April of 1939, she wrote to the finance committee urging that they ask the board to consider relocating both the ICN office and some of its funds to the United States in anticipation of war. Her colleagues were more optimistic than she; they decided that nothing should be done, at least until the office lease expired in 1942. Any decision about the lease became moot when the building was destroyed by bombs in 1941. The ICN's money would remain tied up in Great Britain until the war was over.

So, in July of 1939, while the board dutifully heard reports on Isabel Stewart's survey of graduate education for nurses, the 1941 Congress planned for the United States, and the issue of doing a new history of the ICN, it also discussed what to do about the ICN office in event of war. President Taylor and the staff were empowered by the board to "make the best plans possible." The board also agreed that, if war came, countries able to pay dues should not send them to London but should hold them in abeyance in each country.

## Suspended in War

Before the end of 1939, Poland was overrun, Finland was invaded and the long battle of the Atlantic was underway. The war would drag on for 6 years and eventually permeate every sector of the world. After the July

1939 meeting, no more ICN meetings could be convened until 1944. Acting Executive Secretary Calista Banwarth moved the essential documents of the ICN, first to Cambridge, and then from England to New Haven, Connecticut, USA in October 1939. She later recalled her trepidations setting sail on the S. S. Manhattan: "Besides the general uneasiness . . . as to the dangers of the voyage, my luggage . . . was reported missing. A ten-day trip under these conditions was almost too much for me; but the nervous strain ceased when we sighted New York City and I found Miss Taylor there on the dock to meet me. My recovery was hastened when the thirteen pieces of luggage [containing the ICN materials] were finally brought out of the hold!"[13]

From 310 Cedar Street in New Haven, the dean's office at Yale University School of Nursing, Taylor wrote to all members of the board of directors telling them of what happened and what her plans were. Reminding them that the United States was neutral in the war, she assured the board that the office would be maintained and explained what disposition had been made of ICN property in London. The last issue of *International Nursing Review* was sent out. It would not be published again until 1954. In May 1940, Taylor reluctantly canceled the 1941 Quadrennial Congress planned for Atlantic City, New Jersey. She tried to keep in touch with members by sending messages through nurses newly recruited into the foreign service, the Army Nurse Corps, the Red Cross, or traveling for the Rockefeller Foundation. Years later, she gave much credit to Elizabeth Lind, president of the Swedish Nurses' Association during the war who "was a wonderful medium through whom messages and greetings were forwarded to the nurses in many areas we could not otherwise reach."[14] At the time, there were 32 national associations who were active members of ICN; 7 others were in associated status. Germany and Japan (Italy had

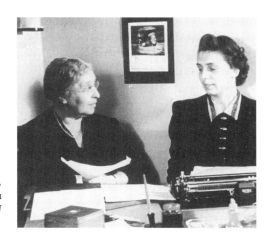

**FIGURE 4-3**
*Effie Taylor, ICN President, 1937 to 1947, with Calista Banwarth in 1942. From AJN Collection.*

left earlier), as well as the countries of eastern Europe, lost contact with the ICN and would remain out of touch for the foreseeable future.

In 1943, Schwarzenberg, now in the United States and finishing studies for her baccalaureate at Columbia University, returned to her post as executive secretary.[15] The next year, when Taylor stepped down as dean at Yale and work for the ICN began to accelerate again, Schwarzenberg set up an ICN office in New York City at 1819 Broadway in space loaned by American nursing organizations.[16]

In October 1944, President Taylor convened an unofficial conference of the ICN at the Henry Hudson Hotel in New York City. In effect, this meeting restarted the ICN as an organization; the participants caught up with wartime events and planned for future board meetings. Most of those who could attend were Americans or Canadians, but, surprisingly, representatives from China, India, Brazil, and New Zealand appeared and a variety of reports from various parts of the world were read or circulated. President Taylor thanked the American Nurses Association for supporting the ICN throughout the war.[17]

## Beginning Again

In spite of its unofficial character, those attending the October meeting discussed a proposed new constitution and by-laws for the ICN and membership rules for the national nursing organizations put forth by Alma Scott, chair of the Constitution and Bylaws Committee. Katherine Densford of Minnesota (USA) moved that the new constitution and bylaws suggestions be sent to countries requesting membership information. The definition of membership in this document read: "All members of this Association shall be nurses, graduates of accredited [state recognized] schools of nursing, which meet the minimum requirements of a nursing school as determined by the ICN."[18] The group decided to circulate this proposal of the committee to national nurse groups interested in applying for membership. Such a definition would have given the ICN remarkable authority over nursing education, but it was never officially adopted. The ICN did reaffirm its traditional policy of recognizing one national organization of nurses in any one country, and continued to insist on self-government by nurses in their member national organizations. These principles would repeatedly be tested in the next decades.

Also on the 1944 meeting agenda was the future of the Florence Nightingale International Foundation (FNIF). American Mary Roberts, chair of the Florence Nightingale Committee of the American Nurses Association (ANA), argued for reorganization of the Foundation. Roberts insisted that Americans would not contribute money to the Foundation unless the FNIF programs "could be understood in terms of the development of nursing in the USA."[19] In what reads like an ultimatum, Roberts

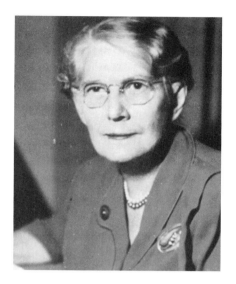

**FIGURE 4-4**
*Mary Roberts, Editor of AJN and activist for postwar changes at ICN. From AJN Collection.*

assured those present that funds for the Foundation would stay with the ANA until a new FNIF plan that appeared reasonable to all was set up. A different proposal called for FNIF to change its status from education to become an administrative/nursing information center housed in London. This was discussed but left dangling. Unspoken but essential to understanding this discussion was the basic question of who would guide the programs of the FNIF, the Americans or the British?

Taylor reported on the ICN plan to communicate through American Army nurses as a way to get in touch with prewar nurse colleagues in occupied countries as soon as the allied armies reached them. This idea was a joint plan relying on cooperation between the ICN and the United Nations Relief and Rehabilitation Administration (UNRRA); when the war was over, the ICN and UNRRA collaborated on assisting displaced nurses who found themselves refugees. Additional discussions of postwar plans for assisting returned military nurses, funding for advanced education, and the problems of staffing hospitals filled the agenda.

The unofficial conference heard a report from Gertrude Pao of China estimating that there were about 8000 nurses in occupied and unoccupied China. She estimated that about 400 nurses graduated each year. Pao described the primitive hospital conditions and problems of war relative to patient care in China's "eighth year of war of resistance against Japanese forces."[20] Reports on nursing from India and South America as well as the United States and Canada included a wealth of detail on economic and educational issues affecting nurses as the war began to draw to a close.

In her history of the period, Daisy Bridges praised Taylor and Banwarth for "indomitable courage and determination" in keeping the ICN alive during the war; she considered its "history unbroken."[21] And, of course, it was crucial that the American Nurses Association spent $71,113.73 to keep ICN going. But, although the ICN held together through the war, it would not be the old ICN that would reemerge or be "resuscitated," as Bridges suggested, but quite a different organization altogether.

In some sense, the March 1947 death of Ethel Fenwick symbolized the transition to an organization more international and less inward looking than in its earlier years. The citation prepared to honor her was read before the assembled 1947 Congress in Atlantic City, New Jersey. Citing Fenwick's crucial role in founding and maintaining the ICN, President Taylor called particular attention to Fenwick's style. "Her penetrating wit and scathing invective were potent weapons in her defense of professional standards of conduct and the salutary discipline upon which they are based never faltered. Loyal throughout her long and brilliant career to the honourable traditions of her native land, she will always remain an example of the steadfastness of mind and spirit which are the pride and glory of the British people. The International Council of Nurses pays affectionate homage to its gallant, farsighted, and indomitable Founder."[22]

## A New Internationalism

"World Health and World Solidarity" combined as the keynote theme of the Ninth ICN Congress when it finally convened at Atlantic City, New Jersey in the United States. This first official postwar meeting resonated with the scope and optimism of the ICN leadership in the immediate postwar era. The first general session developed the theme "Nursing and World Organization in the Fields of Health, Education and Science." A telling indicator of ICN ambitions was the invitation to Brock Chisholm, the new executive secretary of the World Health Organization (WHO), to welcome the participants. Chisholm urged that the ICN and WHO work together, and he forecast an important role for ICN in improving international health.

In sharp contrast to the prewar ICN, the internationalism of 1947 was manifested in a spate of resolutions: to study trade unionism, to support child relief, to support peace via the United Nations, to support the League of the Red Cross, to support international relief work, to urge national professional organizations to engage as economic security spokespersons, and to urge women to become nurses. Sweeping resolutions abounded, and many gained the support of those attending. The new ICN was activist in character and seemed eager to embrace the nationalist-type internationalism of the 1950s.

At least one famous ICN figure was disappointed, however, that the new internationalism of the ICN would not be extended to nurses in

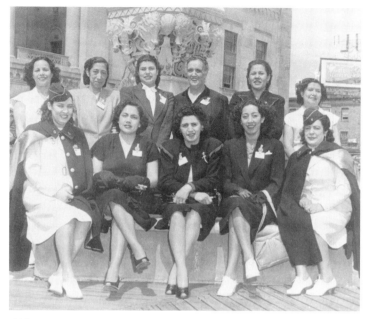

**FIGURE 4-5**
*Group of nurses enjoying the 1947 ICN Congress in Atlantic City,
NJ (USA). From AJN Collection.*

Russia. Lavinia Dock had campaigned in the late 1930s to invite Russian
nurses to participate with the ICN. She tried again to get them invited
to the 1947 meeting. She was deeply disturbed by the barriers between
East and West created by the developing Cold War. Although, at the
time, many others shared her view that the Soviet threat was exaggerated,
the Russian nurses were not invited.[23] Dock, herself, was lauded and feted
as the sole surviving ICN founder and enjoyed the meeting.[24]

Implicit in all this postwar ICN discourse was the assumed superiority
of Anglo-American political institutions and social reforms. Having accepted the recommendations of its "Study of Structure, Functions and
Reorganization" chaired by Alma Scott of the United States, the ICN
mission now would be "to promote the health of nations and to improve
standards of nursing care for the sick, and . . . to assume responsibility for
world leadership in nursing education, not only for the basic and postgraduate education, but also for the education of the nonprofessional
worker."[25] Even as the congress approved its new goals, the ICN leadership
moved to reconfigure its relationship to the FNIF and other international
organizations, especially those in the new United Nations. In 1949, it was
decided that the board of directors of the ICN should act as the Grand

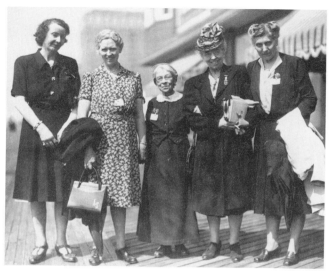

**FIGURE 4-6**

*At the 1947 ICN Congress. Center: Lavinia L. Dock, with Isabel Stewart on her left. Others unidentified. From AJN Collection.*

Council of FNIF. The name of the ICN was changed to International Council of Nurses, With Which is Associated the FNIF.

Gerda Hojer of Sweden was elected the new ICN president at Atlantic City. President Hojer, an experienced educator, studied at the London School of Economics in England and various European countries, including a 1939 fellowship from the Rockefeller Foundation. Born in 1893, and a graduate of the Red Cross nursing school in Stockholm, she spent her early career in various clinical and teaching posts there. In 1934, she

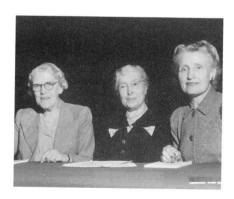

**FIGURE 4-7**

*Mary Lambie (New Zealand) President of FNIP, Effie Taylor, and Katherine Densford President of the American Nurses Association, 1947. From AJN Collection.*

became secretary of the Swedish Nurses Association and was active in the Northern Nurses' Federation and ICN affairs.

Immediately after the congress, plans were made to move the ICN offices back to London. Because of Schwarzenberg's resignation, Virginia Arnold, an American who had been working in Egypt and Greece for UNRRA, took over as acting executive secretary. It was Arnold who, that fall, moved the ICN offices to a bomb-damaged building at 19 Queen's Gate, London. In 1948, Daisy Bridges, formerly associated with the FNIF and a war veteran with the British Army Nursing Service, assumed the post of executive secretary where she would remain for 13 years.

Meanwhile Effie Taylor and Virginia Arnold were actively seeking to forge a strong relationship between WHO and ICN. Historians Richard and Verna Splane describe the first two directors general of WHO, Brock Chisholm and M. G. Candau, as very strong supporters of nursing. In the early debates, they say, it was Irish physician J. D. MacCormack who described the roles played by nurses in health systems around the world. Lucile Petry Leone, chief of the Division of Nursing of the United States Public Health Service, argued for nursing at the first session of the World Health Assembly in Geneva in 1948. She got vital support for this advocacy from her long-time colleague, Thomas Parran, M. D., surgeon general of the United States.[26] Their combined efforts were successful; an official relationship between the ICN and WHO was established in 1948. Virginia Arnold returned to the United States in October of 1948 to accept a position in the United States Public Health Service.[27] Taylor continued her international efforts as an official WHO observer at the United Nations.

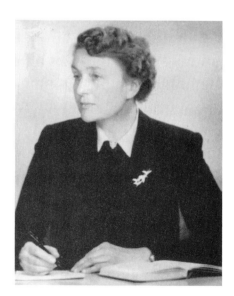

**FIGURE 4-8**
*Daisy Bridges, ICN Executive Secretary, 1948 to 1961. From Bridges, A History of the International Council of Nurses, 1967.*

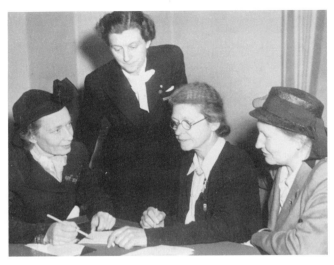

**FIGURE 4-9**
*Ruth Freeman (American Red Cross), Yvonne Hentsch (League of Red Cross Societies), ICN President Gerda Hojer, and FNIP Executive Secretary, Olive Baggaley—1948. From AJN Collection.*

In 1948, Alice Sher joined ICN as assistant general secretary.[28] Sher had been president of the International Nurses Screening Board of UNRRA and later part of the postwar International Refugee Organization (IRO). With her arrival began the special story of the nearly 2000 war refugee nurses who were assisted by ICN between 1950 and 1966. The ICN officially assumed responsibility for the Nurses (Displaced Persons) Professional Register from the IRO in 1950. Alice Sher became the main worker with the refugees. Refugee nurses from the Baltic States, eastern Europe, China, Cuba, Israel, Palestine, Germany, and elsewhere, who were part of the huge refugee migration, sought to verify their nursing credentials and reestablish their careers. The refugee project was vastly complicated by the protracted dislocation caused by the Cold War so that files on the project remained open until 1983.[29]

Continuing complicated issues associated with the so-called exchange of nurses traveling from country to country raised the twin problems of exploitation of traveling nurses and protectionism on the part of nurses in desirable locations. Nurses sought to travel to less ravaged, more affluent postwar countries and requested assistance from ICN. The receiving countries often offered nursing jobs that nurses native to the country would not do. The exchange idea was under constant criticism. In 1953, the Exchange of Nurses Committee, chaired by Margrethe Kruse of Denmark became a standing committee of the ICN.[30]

# An Increasingly Sophisticated ICN

After the ICN offices moved back to London, a larger professional staff and working budget were established; doubling of the dues in 1950 made field work and new program initiatives possible. As noted, the FNIF was absorbed in 1949; ultimately, it became the education arm of the ICN. As Agnes Ohlson would later phrase it, the funds for nursing education would now be spent by the board of ICN. The organization's priorities included professional, social, and economic welfare; nursing education; nursing service (practice); and legislation affecting nursing or nurses. ICN committees began, for the first time, to actually meet face to face instead of doing business by correspondence. In particular, the membership committee assumed a very active role in seeking and reviewing applications from nations in the Middle East, South America, and Africa. By 1957, 46 national associations were active members and 17 countries were in associate status.

Chairman Eli Magnussen's 1953 report to the ICN board described the membership committee's work. Through staff visits and correspondence, they advised national associations on how to meet ICN criteria for joining, then made recommendations of national associations to the board, and later the committee reviewed the status of member countries to ascertain their continued eligibility. Sometimes national associations had to make fairly strenuous efforts to conform to ICN rules. For example, the Nurses' Association of Israel had to solve the question of its relationship to the General Federation of Jewish Labour to prove its independence, and the Japanese had to show how assistant nurses were or were not counted as part of their membership.[31]

The ICN was well positioned to take advantage of post-World War II nationalism because it was, in fact, a federation of national organizations.

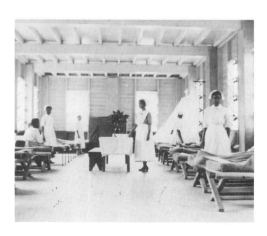

FIGURE 4-10
*Buff Bay Hospital, Jamaica, about 1950. Courtesy Rockefeller Archive Center.*

Immediately after the war was over, a long list of non-European and Third World countries from all sectors of the globe sought admission. By 1957, Haiti, Korea, Turkey, Chile, Jamaica, Luxembourg, Pakistan, Sri Lanka, Trinidad/Tobago, Zambia, Southern Rhodesia, Barbados, Columbia, Ethiopia, Iran, Liberia, Malaya, Panama, Uruguay, Yugoslavia—as well as Italy, Austria, Germany, Israel, and Japan—became new members or rejoined the ICN.

Russia never developed a national nursing organization nor belonged to the ICN. During the existence of the Union of Soviet Socialist Republics, the other members of the Soviet bloc (including some former ICN members) remained outside as well. China joined the ICN in the 1920s under the leadership of Nina Gage and had, throughout invasion, revolution and later the Cultural Revolution, maintained a distinct nursing organization. Although both Peking and the expatriate nurses in Taiwan contacted ICN after World War II, it was Taiwan, persistent in applying for admission, that was rewarded. That decision precluded admission of mainland China during the 1950s.

These effects of the Cold War on the ICN are referred to, in an oblique way, in membership committee reports in 1953. The national nurses' associations of Bulgaria, China, Czechoslovakia, Estonia, Hungary, Poland, Romania, and Yugoslavia were, according to the board of directors, to be "considered inactive for an indefinite period." Kyllikki Pohjala of Finland remarked that the board felt very near the members of the Nurses'

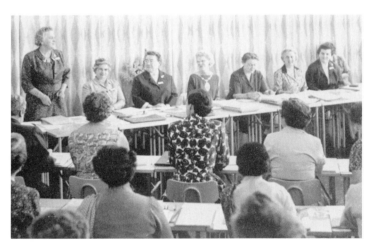

**FIGURE 4-11**

*Kyllikki Pohjala (Finland) speaking to Gladys Schott, Marie Bihet, Agnes Ohlson, Daisy Bridges, Marjorie Marriott and Cercis Jones in Helsinki, 1959. From Bridges, A History of the International Council of Nurses, 1967.*

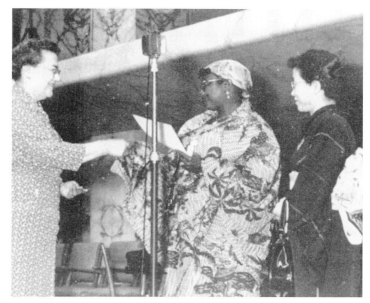

**FIGURE 4-12**
*Marie Bihet, ICN President 1953 to 1957, welcomes Janet Buckle of Liberia accompanied by Shio Hayashi of Japan, 1957. From Bridges, A History of the International Council of Nurses, 1967.*

Association of China and "hoped that the Executive Secretary would keep in close contact with them wherever they were."[32]

On the other hand, nurses in other countries were organizing and gaining new recognition. In Jamaica, for instance, the founding of the Jamaican General Nurses Association in 1946 followed almost immediately on the heels of a new Jamaican Constitution granting universal suffrage. Reforms in the education of nurses and a system of state registration were undertaken by 1951. The Jamaicans applied for and received ICN membership in 1953. The speed and high degree of planning and foresight leading to success in the Jamaican experience symbolized a change in nursing organization in many parts of the world.[33]

## A Host of Issues

Marie Bihet of Belgium was elected ICN president to serve from 1954 to 1957. The long-time director of Brussels' Institute Edith Cavell-Marie DePage, she would preside over an extremely busy and expansive period in the ICN's history. At the ICN, there was heated discussion of the meaning of "socialization" of nursing in countries where national health insurance plans were emerging or changing, as was the case in Canada and Great Britain. In the early 1950s, much concern was also voiced in committee and board meetings about trade unions and their effect on professional associations. A Committee on Economic Welfare and a series of economic consultants collected data on nurses' salaries and working conditions; they offered reports in 1953, 1955, and, most notably, in 1957.[34]

Contacts with the International Labour Organization (ILO) of the United Nations increased, notwithstanding the objections of some members, who feared the taint of labor connections. The ICN and the ILO had a shared history, working together off and on since the time of Secretary Christiane Reimann in the 1920s. When the ILO was reorganized under the United Nations, ICN President Gerda Hojer and others were anxious to take advantage of its data-collecting and recommending powers.

At the 1957 board meeting in Rome, former President Gerda Hojer argued that if the ICN, acting as a professional organization, did not cooperate with ILO, then the question of salaries for nurses might be decided by the trade unions. Denmark's Margrethe Kruse noted that the ILO was a place where workers, employers, and government representatives could collaborate in the cause of social justice. She was selected to lead another study for the ICN on all matters concerning conditions of work and economic aspects of nurses in different countries and prepare conclusions for the ILO Committee on Conditions of Work and Employment of Nurses, then proposed for 1958. At the time, the ILO was investigating work conditions for teachers, journalists, and nurses; it had already made recom-

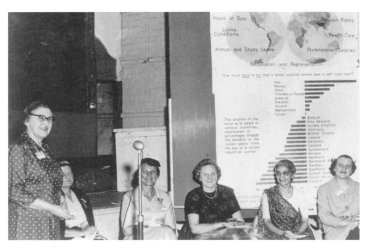

**FIGURE 4-13**
*Florence Udell (UK), reporting for ICN's Social and Economic Welfare Committee, 1961. From AJN Collection.*

mendations to world governments on conditions for manual laborers. In the end, the board agreed that the ICN should apply to be placed on the ILO Special List indicating a consultative relationship.[35] The ICN and ILO worked together cautiously; still, that same year, they mutually agreed that national nurses associations would henceforth be consulted in matters of nurses' economic security.

ICN nurses tried to work out a complex balancing act between those who favored the market-oriented capitalism of the West versus more socialized systems for delivering health care. Many ICN leaders continued their enthusiasm for expanding public health nursing and public health systems in the United States, Finland, Norway, Sweden, Denmark, Brazil, and Germany. But, in spite of supportive rhetoric, not much economic force developed behind the public health reforms proposed immediately after the war. Instead, both in the private sector and in government, the trend was toward investment in rebuilding and creating new acute care institutions.

Responding to the growth in hospital-based nursing, the ICN created a Nursing Service Committee in 1947 and reorganized to create a Division for Nursing Service in 1958. These entities focused on nursing practice and legislation affecting nursing practice that was being proposed in various countries. ICN leaders tried to name the general principles of nursing and clarify nursing's essential role in institutions, in relation to physicians and in determining health policy.

In 1953, an International Code of Ethics was accepted and widely disseminated. The 1953 version acknowledged limitations on nurse authority (ie, the professional nurse was expected to defer to the physician in diagnostic and prescriptive matters).[36] The 1953 Code would later be invoked in the protracted debate on the South African Nurses Association (SANA) and its treatment of colored and black members. In 1965, further changes in the Code reminded nurses of their rights and obligations under the Geneva Conventions of 1949. In 1973, a new code with new language eschewed the idea of physicians as the focus of nurses' loyalty and named the patient as dominant; the nurse's "primary responsibility is to those people who require nursing care."[37]

## Becoming More Truly Universal

During the 1950s and 1960s, the ICN focused its efforts on increasing membership; more participant national associations translated into more dues income. By 1957, the ICN had grown to 43 member countries. Twelve additional national nurse associations were added in 1961: Egypt, Ghana, Guyana, Jordan, Kenya, Mexico, Nigeria, Poland, Singapore, Taiwan, Thailand, and Venezuela. The changing economic and social status of women within these countries, representing mainly African, Asian-

Pacific, and South and Central American regions, was fundamental to the new associations' ability to become ICN members.

Taiwan and Singapore, for example, entered the ranks of the newly industrialized countries in the postwar global market. Singapore, a British colony between 1819 and 1959, was ruled primarily by the People's Action Party (PAP) after the country's independence from Great Britain. PAP encouraged union recruitment of labor and supported the 1961 passage of the Women's Charter, which provided women with "equal pay for equal work."[38] The Singapore Trained Nurses' Association's (STNA), formed in 1957 by a group of senior nurses led by British nurses B. M. Griffin and Edna George and accepted into ICN membership in 1961, represented the successful culmination of nurses' and women's organization, independence, and entry into the country's paid labor market.

African associations underwent a similar transition. Most available accounts of African nursing romanticize rather than address the real struggles of native African women and their attempts to organize their own nursing associations.[39] Written primarily by or about British nurse adventurers in the "dark continent," these "African" accounts illustrate the adventures of white "African Angels" traversing the exotic African terrain as health care missionaries.[40] No doubt this is because, with the exception of Liberia, all sub-Saharan African states were colonial states. The period of colonial rule by European powers—Great Britain, Belgium, France, and Portugal—extended from 1880 to the dissolution of their empires in the 20 years after World War II.[41] France's colonies were primarily in West Africa, Britain's in East and Central Africa, and Portugal's along the coastal areas of East Africa. By 1975, most African states had gained independence from colonial rule.[42]

The combination of World War II and subsequent independence from colonial rule provided an opportunity for changes in the education and employment of women in the African nations more generally and the former British colonies of Egypt, Kenya, Guyana, Ghana, and Nigeria in particular.[43] A British colony since 1884, Nigeria gained independence in 1960. The British system of rules and values generally excluded Nigerian men and women from decision-making responsibilities. Unfortunately, the postindependence government continued gender-based stratification of males to power and women to subordination. Nevertheless, Nigerian women made many important strides toward enhancing their educational and employment opportunities, although clearly never equaling those available to men. By 1960, despite Islamic ideals that minimized women's roles and participation in politics, education, and the paid work force, nurses organized successfully.[44]

The Ghana Registered Nurses Association (GRNA), headed by President and Chief Nursing Officer Miss Docia Kisseih and Vice President Mr. Mettle-Nunoo, was relatively small but well organized when it joined ICN membership in 1961. Like many other African nursing associations, the GRNA had close contact with the ICN and other international agencies for years before its formal association with the ICN. Ethiopia's first nursing school, for example, was started in 1950 by the Ethiopian Red Cross in the Haile Sellasie I Hospital with the assistance of Swedish teachers and materials. At first, students entered the school with only primary school education. Later, the Empress Zewditu Hospital, run by the Seventh Day Adventists, started a nursing school. The Princess Tsehzi Hospital followed in 1952 and later the new St. Paul's Hospital, and the hospital in Asmara. Nursing education and nursing needs in Ethiopia, claimed medical historian Richard Pankhurst, "were adopted as a result of pressure from outside experts and the nursing division of the Ministry of Public Health."[45] As was true in the rest of the world, nursing in Ethiopia developed less with the needs of the home country in mind and more with concern about following Western standards.

But not all African countries with prior international ties became ICN members. Libya signed an agreement with WHO and UNICEF in 1955 to help establish the first school of nursing in the country. The first candidates enrolled in the Tripoli School of Nursing in 1957. The curriculum, taught in Arabic, was modeled on the minimal nurse education requirements established by the ICN, although Libya was not and has never been represented in the ICN.

Nurses in Ghana and other former British colonies in Africa, steeped in British values and traditions, also found ICN ideology more familiar than nurses in either French- or Portuguese-colonized nations. Moreover, many of the former colonies were more economically and socially developed by virtue of their colonial status. But although most Africans in colonized countries were educated by Christian missionaries, secondary education for women was delayed until the 1950s. Hence, many women were ineligible to become nurses under ICN's definition. Expanding educational opportunities ultimately allowed more women access to nursing school admission. However, nursing was still often viewed as "inferior work."[46] Nevertheless, Kenyan Chief Nursing Officer and future ICN President Eunice Muringo Kiereini wrote in 1978, "nursing practice has been and will continue to be influenced by worldwide phenomena or developments and this is even more so in the African continent, where the 'wind of change' is the order of the day."[47]

The acceptance of the Venezuelan and Mexican Nurses' Associations (VNA and MNA) in 1961 followed that of neighboring nursing associations in Brazil (1929), Chile (1953), Colombia (1957), and Uruguay (1957). As was the case in some other Latin American countries, the VNA and MNA were influenced by international entities such as the League of the Red Cross Societies, the Institute of Inter-American Affairs, the W. K. Kellogg Foundation, the Pan American Sanitary Bureau (WHO), and the Rockefeller Foundation.[48]

Although many countries around the world were gaining political independence from colonial rule during the 1960s, others were divided by political takeovers and transitions. Of course, the division of countries

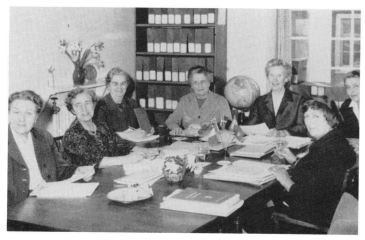

**FIGURE 4-14**

*ICN Membership Committee, 1962. From left: Daisy Bridges, Miss Muntz (Australia), Miss Wright (Canada), ICN President, Mlle Clamageran, Chair of the Membership Committee, Eli Magnussen, Helen Nussbaum and Mlle Rouvier (France). From Bridges, A History of the International Council of Nurses, 1967.*

along political lines yielded consequences for the ICN, especially as the organization attempted to maintain its political neutrality in matters of national politics.

A key example from this period was the application of the Nurses' Association of China (NAC; Taiwan) to ICN membership in 1961. Although NAC's nursing curricula and training standards were well within the established criteria of the ICN Education Committee, the existence of the Nurses' Association of the People's Republic of China (NARCP; Peking), claiming ICN membership since 1922, created a new and complicated situation. Under ICN policy, only one nurse association per country could be recognized and accepted for membership.

Miss Magnussen, chair of the Membership Committee, defended Taiwan's NAC application at the 1961 Board of Directors' meeting in Australia, reasoning that China had been severed into two separate nation states. Hence, she argued, the NAC and the NARCP were nurse associations from two distinct countries. Unable to deal with the political debate surrounding Taiwan's status, the Membership Committee asked NAC to change its name to The Nurses' Association of the Republic of China and resubmit its application as a new country.[49]

Agnes Ohlson, president of the American Nurses Association, was elected ICN president in 1957. Long involved in education and the state regulation of practice, she would be an active and engaged ICN officer.

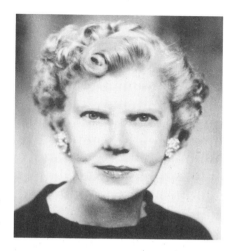

**FIGURE 4-15**
*Agnes Ohlson, ICN President 1957
to 1961. Lynaugh Collection, Bryn
Mawr, PA.*

Attracting more dues-paying members was only a small piece of the ICN's overall agenda for growth and expansion. Indeed, President Ohlson believed nursing needed to expand its confidence along with its geographic influence. Confidence, Ohlson argued, was a key element in educating and communicating the work and worth of nurses around the globe. As she noted in a 1958 *International Nursing Review* editorial,

> In the world today there is a widespread lack of confidence, both in questions of trade and of international politics. It is in this atmosphere, from which none of us can isolate ourselves, that nurses do their daily work of building confidence among those they serve.[50]

## Who Is the Professional Nurse?

As the ICN's growing membership and confidence inflated its ability to "spread nursing's word," more tangible issues related to defining and redefining membership standards were pressing. A 1959 proposal by the Finnish Nurses Association and accepted by the ICN Board of Directors, for example, created stringent admission criteria that mandated general nursing training for nurses from countries already in association or interested in joining the ICN. Many countries protested, arguing that banning specialty-trained nurses from national association membership reduced numbers of eligible nurses, lowered their revenues, and discouraged dues payment to the ICN. The Australian, British, South African, and Northern Rhodesian nursing associations, for example, where many nurses were specialty-trained as midwives, and pediatric and mental health nurses, complained that, if only generalist nurses were accepted into ICN membership, they would likely lose much of their memberships.

Likewise, large numbers of mental health and tuberculosis nurses in The National Association of Trained Nurses in France jeopardized the association's standing in the ICN. In echoed concern, Hong Kong, Singapore, Kenya, and Trinidad argued that nurse training reflected "the needs of their community" and that the new ICN membership criteria were in opposition to their country's fundamental nursing needs.[51] Indian nurse Dr. Marie Jahoda, whose country's tuberculosis nurses were the principal caregivers to escalating numbers of tubercular patients, warned the ICN that "international policies and international actions are only possible if one does not deny the differences in identity of various nations and the differences in the problems they face."[52]

Responding to myriad complaints from member countries about the new specialist-generalist requirements, the ICN Board rescinded the 1959 proposal in 1961. Later the same year, however, the Grand Council adopted a new principle for membership mandating that national nurses' associations seeking ICN membership be "composed exclusively of professional nurses." Professional nurses were defined as those who had "completed generalised nursing preparation in an approved school of nursing and [were] authorised to practice nursing in their country." Acknowledging that generalist preparation was not the standard for every country in ICN membership, the report concluded that only nurses who graduated during or after 1965 would be expected to have such preparation.[53] Although ICN leaders agreed to accept specialty-trained nurses into membership temporarily, their clear objective was that future ICN membership would require generalist training. The longstanding specialist-generalist debate seemed an unending source of controversy. The Hong Kong Nurses and Midwives Association (HKNMA), for example, met with ICN Director of Nursing Services Frances Beck in 1961 to discuss the association's potential but problematic membership with the ICN. The problem with accepting HKNMA into ICN membership was the association's joint membership of nurses and midwives, because the latter were not trained nurses. Beck informed the HKNMA that, to meet ICN eligibility criteria, the non-nurse midwives would need to be reclassified as "associate" rather than full association members. The association's midwives found their reclassification unacceptable and refused to support the HKNMA's bid for ICN membership. Other trained nurses in the HKNMA, especially expatriate nurses working in the Hong Kong government service, joined the midwives in protest. The split in HKNMA ranks led Beck to suggest that interested HKNMA nurse members form a new association, rename it the Hong Kong Nurse's Association, and apply for ICN membership separately.[54] Taking her advice, a subcommittee organized the Hong Kong Nurses' Association (HKNA) in August 1961; by March 1964, the HKNA was formed with 533 nurse members and was accepted into ICN membership at the 13th Quadrennial ICN Congress in Frankfurt, Germany in June 1965.[55] The specialist-generalist issue was, in a more broad sense, a competing wedge between the ICN's professionalizing ideology and the day-to-day realities of nursing education and practice in individual countries. Indeed, some extensively educated generalist-trained nurses, although members of the ICN sisterhood, could actually be viewed as outsiders within their own countries. Insisting on generalist nurse training in less industrialized countries, where limited educational opportunity and great public health problems seemed to justify more quickly trained nurses, emphasized the ICN creed of high international nursing education standards over quick solutions to national health problems.

## Defining Nursing Around the World

Finding a universal, shared definition of nursing was an elusive objective of the ICN throughout the postwar period. As we have seen, a series of questions plagued the definition makers. Must the nurse be a generalist first or could nurses trained only in specialty fields meet the definition? Should midwives be included? How should trained nurses relate to assistant nurses? And, finally, the most vexing question of all: what scope of professional authority should be held by the nurse? Back in 1929, a footnote was added to the ICN Constitution defining the nurse as "someone who was instructed in at least four of the main branches of nursing . . . and prepared upon graduation to enter general practice of nursing." This proved unworkable because, at that time, basic training limited to a specialty was commonly accepted for state nurse registration in many countries. The definition prepared for the 1961 Congress in Melbourne, Australia stipulated that nurses were prepared to care for " . . . people of all ages in the promotion of health and in all forms of sickness both physical and mental."[56] This formulation was not acceptable to the congress either.

Two years earlier, however, in 1959, the ICN approved publication of *Basic Principles of Nursing Care* by Virginia Henderson of the United States. This little 50-page pamphlet, reprinted six times in the next decade, became a best seller and guide in 12 languages. Henderson's intent was to describe the care "that any person requires no matter what the physician's diagnosis and the therapy he prescribes although both influence the plan she initiates and carries out . . . the nurses basic care is the same whether the patient is considered physically or mentally ill."[57] She insisted she was discussing all settings and that the same principles applied in both preventive and curative nursing.

What captured the imagination of those who read her book was Henderson's idea of the essential or unique function of the nurse. She offered her own concept in the absence of a shared international

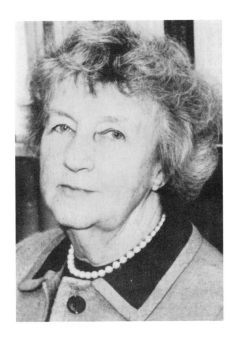

**FIGURE 4-16**
*Virginia Henderson (USA). From AJN Collection.*

definition. "The unique function of the nurse is to assist the individual, sick or well, in the performance of those activities contributing to health or its recovery (or to a peaceful death) that he would perform unaided if he had the necessary strength, will or knowledge. It is likewise her function to do this in such a way as to help him gain independence as rapidly as possible."[58]

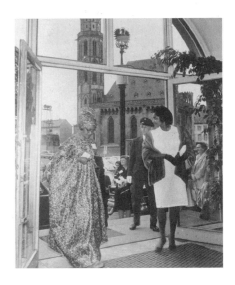

**FIGURE 4-17**
*Delegates arriving at ICN Congress in Frankfurt, 1965. From AJN Collection.*

Finally, in 1965, the ICN Congress in Frankfurt, Germany was able to agree on two definitions. "The nurse is a person who has completed a programme of basic nursing education and is qualified and authorized in her country to supply the most responsible service of a nursing nature for the promotion of health, the prevention of illness and the care of the sick." And, for nursing education, "Basic nursing education is a planned educational programme which provides a broad and sound foundation for the effective practice of nursing and a basis for advanced nursing education."[59] Of course, that was not the end of it; the definition of nursing would be revisited in each decade to follow.

## Human Rights and Nursing

After World War II, South African apartheid policies and particularly the 1957 South African Nursing Amendment Act institutionalized social and spatial barriers between black, white, and colored nurses and their patients. Authority relations inscribed in South African law decreed that only whites could hold leadership positions or represent nursing interests on either national or international policy-making bodies. The 1957 Nursing Act further elaborated the caste system by making it illegal for black nurses, however senior, to give orders to white nurses, however junior.[60]

At the ICN, various countries raised questions about the effect of racial segregation policies in South Africa. They especially questioned the effect of the South African Nursing Act of 1957 on the status of African and "colored" nurses in SANA. In 1959, the racial segregation issue was forced into debate by India and Sweden. "Resolved, that the ICN be asked to request its member associations to ensure that no qualified nurse is debarred from . . . full membership of her national association on grounds of race, religion or color."[61]

Defending her association, South Africa's M. G. Borcherds used the ICN's own apolitical argument and rhetoric, "[It is] my great regret that in a nonpolitical organization such as this claims to be, a member country could make an attack on the integrity of another member country."[62] Borcherds' strategy was effective and the ICN did back off. Moreover, initial criticism of SANA's practices were reversed when the ICN celebrated the SANA's Golden Jubilee in November 1964 and awarded the John Tremble medal to SANA President Charlotte Searle for her role in passing the 1944 South African Nursing Act (Nursing Act No. 45).[63] Although the ICN Board's attitude toward SANA's racially biased policies and practices was ambivalent and contradictory, historian Shula Marks credits the ICN's questioning with the prevention of even more radically discriminative measures such as the adoption of differential nursing standards, uniforms, and insignias between nonwhite and white nurses.[64]

Of course, the United States just barely avoided becoming the target of similar criticism by restructuring its professional organizations and including black nurses in ANA membership in 1952. South Africa continued to defend its policies on the grounds that national nurse associations had the right of self-determination. However, the finding that SANA was not free from dictation of its policies by the South African government undermined their defense. The issue came up again and again, and, finally, South Africa was forced to withdraw from ICN.

## New Leaders Coping With Old Problems

The ICN's sixth decade began with new leadership. In 1961, French nurse Alice Clamageran succeeded Agnes Ohlson as ICN president. Clamageran began her professional nursing career at the Red Cross School of Nursing in Rouen and later studied at London's Bedford College as a Florence Nightingale scholar before earning her public health nursing certificate at the University of London. After completion of her London-based education, Clamageran returned to France and was elected president of the National Association of Trained Nurses of France (NATNF) in 1950.[65]

Helene Nussbaum assumed the general secretary position when Daisy Bridges retired in 1961. A Swiss citizen born in Sicily, Nussbaum trained with the Italian Red Cross in Naples and later obtained her Swiss graduate nurse diploma. Conversant in English, French, Italian, German, and modern Greek, Nussbaum held a variety of positions under the sponsorship

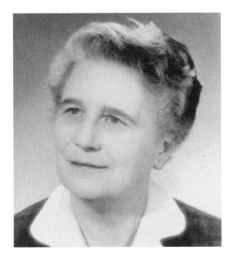

FIGURE 4-18
Alice Clamageran, ICN President 1961 to 1965. From AJN Collection.

of UNRRA, WHO, and the International Committee of the Red Cross (ICRC). Returning to Geneva in 1958, Nussbaum was appointed executive secretary of the Swiss Association of Graduate Nurses, a position she held until her appointment as ICN general secretary.[66]

As this new but experienced leadership took hold, the ICN encountered a familiar problem. Holding the ICN membership together despite national differences was crucial to meeting the ICN's pressing financial needs. Unpaid or late membership dues were a constant concern, particularly because they constituted the main source of revenue. In 1963, for example, membership dues accounted for £57,082 of £63,470 income for the year.[67] The remaining income was generated by subscription charges for the *International Nursing Review* and publication sales, interest and dividends, and private donations. By 1969, dues still represented over 80% of the organization's income, a fact that propelled the Finance Committee to engage in "vigorous correspondence" with countries to encourage timely payments.[68] The Burma Nurses Association and the Federation of Nurses Associations of Yugoslavia, for example, were contacted repeatedly about their payments in arrears in 1969. The persistent persuasion used to remind associations to pay up was reported to have made "the total [financial] situation a great deal better."[69]

Reflecting on her 4-year tenure as ICN president (1961–1965), Alice Clamageran summed up the years' most important changes as the "improvement in relationships," the "exchange of ideas," and "better contact."[70] The ICN's communication campaign included over 30 national associations field-visited by nurse advisors, whereas the Newsletter sent news from headquarters to national associations every 2 months. President Clamageran believed these efforts improved relationships with other international organizations, dialogue between ICN national nurses' associations, and rapport among individual ICN committee members.[71]

Indeed, when Canadian Alice Girard assumed her presidential duties in 1965, the ICN still stressed the concept of communication throughout almost all of its activities.[72] As thousands of nurses gathered in Frankfurt, Germany for the 1965 Quadrennial Congress, they were reminded of the ICN's new organizing framework through the Congress' "Communication" theme. Keynote speaker Magda Kelber examined the role of communication as the ICN's overarching paradigm. Answering her own question, "Does [the theme] imply that communication will automatically eliminate conflict, and that conflict should be eliminated?," Kelber argued that communication played a key role in eradicating differences between conflicting points of view by "clarifying disagreements, analysing the reasons for them, sifting real from apparent controversy, and helping [us] recognise our hidden and often unconscious motivations," thus turning "destructive conflict into constructive controversy."[73]

The ICN had finally resumed publication of the *International Nursing Review* in 1957, after an 18-year hiatus. Marjorie Wenger, the former

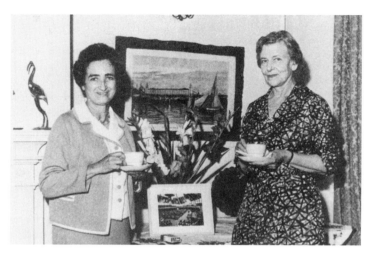

**FIGURE 4-19**
*Alice Girard, ICN President 1965 to 1969, with Helen Nussbaum,
ICN General Secretary 1961 to 1967. From ICN Collection.*

editor of *Nursing Times,* was hired as the journal's first full-time editor. She was charged with increasing journal circulation and publishing six issues a year, up from its previous quarterly distribution. The reinstated *International Nursing Review* provided a means to exchange, compare, and contrast professional concerns, events, ideas, and care technologies among countries. Between 1958 and 1970, the *International Nursing Review* focused on ICN headquarter activities, worldwide health care problems, and innovations in health care delivery. ICN staff changes, visits to headquarters by dignitaries and other nursing leaders, and biographic sketches of ICN leaders comprised much of the "ICN News."

Wenger increased *International Nursing Review* subscriptions from 2162 in 1961 to 2543 in 1964 before her resignation in December 1964.[74] After 1970, with new editor Alice Thompson in place, the *International Nursing Review* reflected shifting concerns among nurses dealing with issues of professionalization, education, image, physician/nurse collaboration, new nursing roles, and research. ICN historian Daisy Bridges congratulated the journal for "bringing before related organizations and the general public a true picture of the nurses' contribution to the health and well-being of the community."[75]

One of the ICN's most significant acts in the 1960s was the board of directors' decision to relocate ICN headquarters from London back to Geneva. The move, the board thought, would enable the ICN to "move in the same circles" with other international organizations and maintain its place as nursing's global representative. The board was concerned that without a physical presence in matters related to nursing, the ICN and nursing would

## THEMES OF INTERNATIONAL NURSES DAY

The ICN created the idea of International Nurses Day (IND) in 1965. May 12th, Florence Nightingale's birthday, was chosen as the day of celebration. A theme reflecting ICN goals is set each year.

| | |
|---|---|
| 1971 | Unity |
| 1972 | Nurses' Role in Policy Making |
| 1973 | The Nurses' Role in Safeguarding the Human Environment |
| 1974 | Code for Nurses—Ethical Concepts Applied to Nursing |
| 1975 | International Women's Year |
| 1976 | Know Your Nurse |
| 1977 | The Nurse as an Instrument of Change |
| 1978 | Better Conditions for Nurses—Key to Better Health Care |
| 1979 | International Year of the Child |
| 1980 | The Role of Nursing in Primary Health Care |
| 1981 | United Nations International Year of Disabled Persons |
| 1982 | World Assembly on the Aging |
| 1983 | Practice and People: Nurses' Role in Primary Health Care |
| 1984 | Nurses Speak Up for Better Health |
| 1985 | End of the UN Decade for Women—Nurses and Women's Health—One Step Towards Happier Families |
| 1986 | Immunization for All the World's Children |
| 1987 | Health in the Workplace |
| 1988 | Safe Motherhood |
| 1989 | School Health |
| 1990 | Nurses and the Environment |
| 1991 | Mental Health—Nurses in Action |
| 1992 | Healthy Aging |
| 1993 | Quality, Costs and Nursing |
| 1994 | Healthy Families for Healthy Nation |
| 1995 | Women's Health—Nurses Pave the Way |
| 1996 | Better Health Through Nursing Research |
| 1997 | Healthy Young People = A Brighter Future |
| 1998 | Partnership for Community Health |
| 1999 | Celebrating Nursing's Past, Claiming the Future |
| 2000 | Nurses—Always There for You |

be misrepresented by other groups. Citing an incident in which UNESCO listed the ICN as a "woman's organization," the board demonstrated that only after vigorous protest by the ICN did UNESCO reclassify the ICN among the "Organizations of Natural Sciences."[76] The ICN, of course, had already established working relationships with other international bodies in Geneva from its London-based office. Indeed, ICN representatives created an ICN "presence" among a wide array of international organizations, including the United Nations, UNICEF, the World Health Organization, the League of Red Cross Societies, the International Confederation of Midwives, the International Labor Office, the International Hospital Federation, the World Medical Association, the World Federation for Mental Health, the International Union of Health Education, and the International Committee of Catholic Nurses and Social Workers.[77] Nevertheless, advocates for the move argued that continuation of an ICN presence depended on closer geographic proximity to other international bodies.

The move to Geneva underscored the ICN's new expanded communication agenda while raising a host of relevant questions. Given the ICN's perennial financial concerns, was it cost-effective to move the organization? Did the advantages of moving outweigh the move's financial investment? Given that the Florence Nightingale International Foundation was required by decree to remain in London, would splitting the ICN's educational arm from the central organizational body have an adverse effect on the ICN's educational agenda? Could the ICN afford *not* to move?

After a thorough analysis of both the economic and noneconomic concerns of ICN leaders, consultant Brech concluded that relocating ICN headquarters to Geneva was both-cost effective and more consistent with the ICN's externalizing agenda.[78] Based on his recommendation, the ICN established a new headquarters in Geneva in 1966, although many of the London-based staff remained behind.

## At Seventy

As the ICN moved toward greater organizational strength, its leaders focused their efforts on uniting and enlarging their involvement in global nursing matters. Postwar changes in health care and health priorities forced them to reexamine and redefine nursing. The ICN tried to explain and defend nursing's work worldwide and claimed its place as nursing's voice in an ever-widening circle of influence. This broad organizational self-concept stood in sharp contrast with the more modest scope of earlier ICN concerns about nursing education and practice. As the ICN focused its efforts outward, however, it faced escalating challenges balancing and financing its new agenda while, at the same time, maintaining internal cohesion in the face of political upheaval, economic fluctuations, and divisive racial and gender conflicts.

## ENDNOTES

1. Minutes, ICN Board of Directors, London, July 1937, ICNA. The first executive secretary of the ICN, Christiane Reimann, announced her resignation in 1933 but stayed with the ICN until June 1934, spending 2 weeks with her successor, Anna Schwarzenberg. Then she left on holiday. In July, Treasurer Ellen Musson and Dame Lloyd Still went to Geneva. They asked Reimann to return and meet with them, but she declined. Reimann planned to edit the *International Nursing Review* as recommended in the internal reorganization plan for the ICN. Possibly for reasons of ill health or perhaps because Lloyd Still did not approve, Reimann did not become editor. She formally resigned all posts in October 1934. During her 12 years with the ICN, Reimann often paid its expenses out of her own pocket. Her socialist views often conflicted with the more conservative Ethel Bedford Fenwick.

2. Anna Schwarzenberg obviously felt very cut off in Geneva and complained of the difficulty in obtaining and retaining staff. She also worried about "serious disturbance in Europe" and its effect on communications and the flow of funds. Minutes, International Council of Nurses, Board of Directors, London, July 1937, ICNA.

3. Australia's associations formed in sequence (ie, Australian Trained Nurses Association [1899] in New South Wales, followed by Queensland, South Australia, West Australia, and Tasmania). The Royal Victorian Trained Nurses' Association was founded in 1901; the associations formed the Australian Nursing Federation in 1904.

4. Proceedings, International Council of Nurses, Eighth Congress, London, 1937, p. 46, ICNA.

5. Minutes, Grand Council, London, 1937, ICNA.

6. Ibid.

7. Proceedings, Eighth Congress, London 1937, p. 13, ICNA.

8. Bridges, 107.

9. International Council of Nurses, Eighth Congress, National Reports, London, 1937, p. 13, ICNA.

10. Hilde Steppe, "Historical Research in Nursing," *Proceedings Volume,* Workgroup of European Nurse Researchers, Fifth Biennial Conference, September 1990, p. 310.

11. Frau Oberin Blunck, Minutes, International Council of Nurses, Board of Directors, London, July 1939, ICNA. Frau Blunck survived the war to see partial restoration of her national nursing organization; she died in 1947.

12. President's Address, International Council of Nurses, Board of Directors, London, July 1939, ICNA.

13. Bridges, 116.

14. Effie Taylor, "The Past is Inspiring," *International Nursing Review* (July 1959): 28. Jean I. Gunn, the ICN's first vice president, on whom Taylor relied for consultation often during this difficult period, unfortunately died at age 59 of cancer in June 1941.

15. Effie Taylor arranged with Mary Beard, director of nursing service for the American Red Cross, to give a study scholarship to Schwarzenberg for a year of study at Columbia. Taylor, *International Nursing Review* (July 1959): 29.

16. The ICN offices shared a building with the National Council for War Defense, a board of leaders of American nursing organizations set up to recruit nurses for the war effort and expand the number of nurses available for civilian caregiving.

17. In her 1967 history, Bridges reports that the 1944 unofficial meeting did not take place, but it did. The first official meeting of the board of directors was convened in London in 1946.

18. Minutes, unofficial conference of the International Council of Nurses, New York, October 6 and 7, 1944, p. 11, ICNA.
19. Ibid., p. 16.
20. Report from Gertrude Pao, Annex 7, unofficial ICN board meeting, New York, 1944, ICNA. See also Kaiyi Chen, "Quality Versus Quantity."
21. Bridges, 123.
22. "In Memoriam, Ethel Gordon Fenwick," International Council of Nurses, Proceedings, Ninth Congress, Atlantic City, NJ, 1947, ICNA.
23. See Norman Davies, *A History of Europe* (Oxford and New York: Oxford University Press, 1996) for a discussion of the American Truman Doctrine of Containment, the Berlin Blockade, and the rapidly emerging East–West schism in 1947 and 1948.
24. Lavinia Dock died in April 1956.
25. The complete name of Scott's committee was Study of the Structure, Functions and Reorganization of the ICN as Well as Its Relationships with Other Organizations. Minutes, International Council of Nursing, Board of Directors, Brussels, Belgium, 1951, ICNA. For quote see, Gerda Hojer, President's Address, International Council of Nurses, Board of Director's Meeting, London, 1948, ICNA.
26. Richard and Vera Splane, *Chief Nursing Officer Positions in National Ministries of Health* (San Francisco, CA: The Regents University of California, 1994), 135, 162.
27. In 1954, WHO announced that the theme for World Health Day would be "nursing."
28. Quinn, *ICN Past and Present,* 16.
29. Alice C. Sher, "The Stranger in Our Midst," *International Nursing Review,* 7 (October 1960): 11–17.
30. Barbara L. Brush, "'Exchangees' or Employees? The Exchange Visitor Program and Foreign Nurse Immigration to the United States, 1945–1990," *Nursing History Review,* 1 (1993): 171–180.
31. For two recent historical studies describing some of the issues confronted in the postwar world by nurses seeking to establish nursing education and professional standards, see Colleen E. Bowers, "Passing the Lamp: The Status and Conditions of Nursing in Pakistan at the Time of Independence," and Reiko Shimazaki Ryder and Tosiko Yamada, "The Policy of American Occupation and Its Influence on Nursing in Japan, 1945–1951." Both papers were presented at the 14th Annual Conference of the American Association for the History of Nursing, September 26–28, 1997, Hartford, CT, USA.
32. International Council of Nurses, Minutes, Membership Committee Report, Grand Council, San Paulo, Brazil, 1953, ICNA.
33. "The Story of the 25 Years," *The Jamaican Nurse,* 11 (August 1971): 8, 9, and 11.
34. Report of the Economic Consultant, International Council of Nurses, Board of Directors, Rome, Italy, 1957, ICNA. This is an interesting document based on data provided by "economic consultants" from 21 countries who supplied information on salaries, hours of work, rank and status, vacation, and other benefits. The "consultants" seem to have been nurses who were willing to solicit whatever information they could and share it with ICN. All this probably helped the ICN discuss the issues, but, as the consultants themselves conceded, there was not enough quality information on which any recommendations could be based.
35. Minutes, International Council of Nurses, Board of Directors, Rome, Italy, 1957, ICNA.
36. International Code of Nursing Ethics, The Grand Council of the International Council of Nurses, San Paulo, Brazil, 1953, ICNA. It begins: "Professional nurses minister to the sick, assume responsibility for creating a physical, social and spiritual environment

which will be conducive to recovery, and stress the prevention of illness and promotion of health by teaching and example. They render health service to the individual, the family, and the community and coordinate their services with members of other health professions.

Service to mankind is the primary function of nurses and reason for the existence of the nursing profession. Need for nursing service is universal. Professional nursing service is therefore unrestricted by considerations of nationality, race, creed, colour, politics or social status.

Inherent in the code is the fundamental concept that the nurse believes in the essential freedoms of mankind and the preservation of human life.

The profession recognizes that an international code cannot cover in detail all the activities and relationships of nurses, some of which are conditioned by personal philosophies and beliefs."

The Code then goes on to outline 14 specific responsibilities for nurses, including 3 that refer to deference and support for physicians and 3 on appropriate personal conduct.

37. Minutes, International Council of Nurses, Board Meeting, Mexico City, 1973, ICNA.
38. Janet W. Saleff, "Women, the Family, and the State: Hong Kong, Taiwan, Singapore—Newly Industrialized Countries in Asia," in Sharon Stichter and Jane L. Parpart, Eds. *Women, Employment and the Family in the International Division of Labour* (Philadelphia: Temple University Press, 1990), 98–136.
39. See, for example, Dea Birkett, "The White Woman's Burden," in Chaudhuri and Strobel, Eds., *Western Women and Imperialism*, 177–188.
40. Bridget M. Robertson's *Angels in Africa: A Memoir of Nursing With the Colonial Service* (London: The Radcliffe Press, 1993) is a good example. Robertson, a member of the Queen Elizabeth Overseas Nursing Service, describes her exploits through Kenya, Kilifi, the Seychelles Islands, Nigeria, and Kenya in the 1950s. Although she makes reference to native practices (ie, Muslim women in purdah in Kenya), the book focuses on her personal experiences.
41. Lynne Brydon and Sylvia Chant, *Women in the Third World: Gender Issues in Rural and Urban Areas* (New Brunswick, NJ: Rutgers University Press, 1989), 33. See also Davies, *A History of Europe*.
42. The conflict in Southern Rhodesia (Zimbabwe) continued until 1980.
43. The two previous African nurses' associations in membership, Zambia and Ethiopia, joined in 1953 and 1957, respectively.
44. Jane L. Parpart, "Wage Earning Women and the Double Day: The Nigerian Case," in Stichter and Parpart, Eds. *Women, Employment, and the Family,* 161–182. Females comprised only 37% of the primary students, 18% of the secondary school students, and 7% of students in postsecondary institutions in Nigeria at the time.
45. See Richard Pankhurst, *An Introduction to the Medical History of Ethiopia* (Trenton, NJ: The Red Sea Press, Inc., 1990), 255–260, for a brief discussion of nursing in Ethiopia.
46. Hilda Hakim, "Tripoli School of Nursing, Libya, North Africa," *International Nursing Review*, 7, (December 1960): 39–42; Lyle Creelman, "Nursing in the African Region," *International Nursing Review*, 5, (April 1958): 19–20. Creelman reviews nursing in various African countries and notes that in Zanzibar "girls find teacher training more attractive than nurse training" (p. 20).
47. Eunice Muringo Kiereini, "What's New in Nursing Practice: Africa," *The Jamaican Nurse*, 18 (April/May 1978): 25.
48. Abu-Saad, *A World View*, 110–122.

49. Minutes, International Council of Nurses, Board of Directors, Wellington, New Zealand, 10–12 April 1961, p. 29, ICNA. Treasurer Marjorie Marriot asked Miss Magnussen if the same would apply to North Korea and East Germany if they applied for membership. Magnussen said that it would.

50. "Editorial," *International Nursing Review*, 5, (January 1958): 3.

51. Minutes, International Council of Nurses, Board of Directors, Wellington, New Zealand, 10–12 April 1961, p. 32, ICNA.

52. Marie Jahoda, "Resume of Congress," *The Nursing Journal of India*, 52, (August 1961): 215.

53. Minutes, International Council of Nurses, Grand Council, "Progress Report on an Inquiry Into Basic Nursing Education, 1961–1963," Melbourne, Australia, 17–19 April 1961, p. 1, ICNA.

54. Miss Frances S. Beck, "Notes on a Visit to Hong Kong," November 1961, Country Files (Hong Kong), pp. 1–5, ICNA.

55. See Elaine Y. W. Poon, "The Formation of the Hong Kong Nurses Association," *The Hong Kong Nursing Journal*, 3 (May 1967): 73–74 and Sheila Iu, "President's Address," *The Hong Kong Nursing Journal*, 9 (November 1970): 3–9. The Hong Kong Nurses and Midwives Association became the Hong Kong Midwives Association shortly after the HKNA was accepted into ICN membership.

56. Quinn, 26.

57. Virginia Henderson, *Basic Principles of Nursing Care* (Basel, Switzerland: S. Karger, 1969), 1.

58. Henderson, 50.

59. Bridges, 223–224.

60. For the complete history, see Marks, *Divided Sisterhood*. Marks notes that the original act made it illegal for black physicians to give orders to white nurses, however this clause was eventually deleted.

61. Minutes, International Council of Nurses, Board of Directors, Helsinki, Finland, 1959, ICNA.

62. Minutes, International Council of Nurses, Board of Directors, Wellington, New Zealand, 10–12 April 1961, p. 40, ICNA. The SANA deliberation was dropped afterwards.

63. "Celebrating the First Fifty Years: The South African Nursing Association," *International Nursing Review*, 12 (January/February 1965): 7–8. John Tremble, a London-trained physician, is credited with founding the first South African nursing journal, *The South African Nursing Record*, in 1913 and the South African Trained Nurses Association (SATNA) in 1914. See Marks, *Divided Sisterhood*, 62.

64. Marks, *Divided Sisterhood*, 185.

65. "Alice Clamageran, President ICN," *International Nursing Review*, 8 (July/August 1961): 71.

66. "Introducing Helene Nussbaum," *International Nursing Review*, 7 (August 1960): 2–4; "Helene Nussbaum: Executive Director International Council of Nurses, 1961–1967," *International Nursing Review*, 14 (July/August 1967): 5; Alice Clamageran, "A Tribute to Helen Nussbaum," *International Nursing Review*, 14 (July/August 1967): 6–7.

67. The United States paid 20,917, followed by Canada's 8,102, Great Britain and Northern Ireland's 5,868, and Japan's 2,940, all paid in pounds sterling(£). Minutes, International Council of Nurses, Council of National Representatives, Geneva, December 31, 1963, Accounts, Agenda Item 10, Annex 3, pp. 1–3, ICNA.

68. Minutes, International Council of Nurses, Board of Directors, 18–20 June 1969, Montreal, Canada, Agenda Item 9, *To Receive Information on the Situation as Regards Nonpayment of Dues by Certain Member Associations*, p. 10. ICNA.

69. After the ICN headquarters moved to Geneva in 1966, budget figures are reported in Swiss francs. In 1969, 730,000 francs in dues were collected with a total income of 812,000. International Council of Nurses, Council of National Representatives, Financial Report, Montreal, Canada, June 1969, Agenda Item 7, Annex IX, p. 6, ICNA.

70. "Messages From Former ICN Presidents," Alice Clamageran, *International Nursing Review*, 21 (1974): 80.

71. "Report of the ICN President, Alice Clamageran, 1961–1965," *International Nursing Review*, 12 (May/June 1965): 11.

72. Girard was the ICN's first Canadian President. For an interesting biography of Alice Girard, see Alice Caplin, "Alice A. Girard: Canada's Premier Nurse," *Proceedings of the Canadian Association for the History of Nursing*, Third Annual Conference, Calgary, 27–28 June 1990.

73. Magda Kelber, "Communication or Conflict," Congress Keynote Address, International Council of Nurses, 13th Quadrennial Congress, Frankfurt, Germany, 21 June 1965. Reprinted in *International Nursing Review*, 12 (May/June 1965): 29–36.

74. Helen Nussbaum, "Report of the ICN General Secretary," *International Nursing Review*, 12 (May/June 1965): 20.

75. Daisy C. Bridges, "'*International Nursing Review*': Past, Present and Progress," *International Nursing Review*, 15 (January 1968): 14. The first ICN publication was the *The ICN* (Bulletin) circulated at intervals between 1922 and 1925 at Christiane Reimann's personal expense. From 1926 to 1929, the publication was named *The ICN* and was published quarterly. Renamed *International Nursing Review* in 1929, the journal was published six times yearly between 1929 and 1939 until World War II added to its financial difficulties, which forced termination.

76. Minutes, International Council of Nurses, Board of Directors, Wellington, New Zealand, 10–11 April 1961, ICNA. The ICN made clear to UNESCO that they represented thousands of male nurses as well.

77. Minutes, International Council of Nurses, Board of Directors, Frankfurt/Main, Federal Republic of Germany, 13–15 June 1965,: 35–38, ICNA.

78. Minutes, International Council of Nurses, Board of Directors, Frankfurt/Main, Federal Republic of Germany, 13–15 June 1965, E. F. L. Brech, "The Future Location of ICN Headquarters," Annex 5, pp. 19–20, ICNA.

# F I V E

# New Missions, New Meanings

## BARBARA L. BRUSH

*I*n 1969, Alice Girard relinquished charge of an inexperienced staff to incoming President Margrethe Kruse. Of the six staff members at the new ICN headquarters, only Sheila Quinn and nurse advisor Martha "Biddy" Shout had been employed for more than 3 years; the other nurse advisors and office support staff had been there less than a year.

Kruse, whose strong economic focus stemmed from 27 years as executive secretary of the Danish Nurses' Organization (DNO; 1945–1972), 13 years as chairperson of the ICN Committee on Exchange of Privileges for Nurses (EPN), and 4 years on the Social and Economic Welfare Committee (SEW), worried that the organization's low salaries and high work demands would create more staff turnover.[1] Concerned particularly about losing its most senior staff, Kruse reported to the board of directors: "I have known for a long time that Biddy Shout thought of resigning because she felt that she could not continue on the low salary level for her remaining working life . . . .Now I have *asked* [Kruse's emphasis] her to stay and told her that at the next Board of Directors meeting I shall suggest a revision of the salary scales."[2]

Kruse understood Shout's worth as a liaison between the ICN and its new African member associations. As the former principal nursing tutor and registrar of the Nurses Board of Ghana, Shout was well acquainted with the African territories.[3] With increasing membership critical to its survival, the ICN could ill afford to lose the expertise of one of its most experienced staff members.

But almost as soon as Kruse took office, Executive Director Sheila Quinn announced her resignation to accept a chief nursing officer position in England.[4] Kruse quickly looked for a suitable replacement. The ideal candidate, as advertised among ICN member organizations and the professional press, would be active in his/her national nurse association, fluent in English with a working knowledge of French, knowledgeable about nursing education and general nursing development, and experienced in leadership and management. Former Deputy Executive Director of the American Nurses Association, Adele Herwitz, agreed to serve as interim director in March 1970 until such a person could be found.

By May 1970, four people had applied for the post. It became apparent, however, that Kruse had Herwitz in mind for the ICN's top management

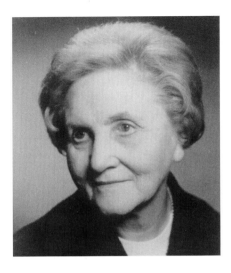

**FIGURE 5-1**
*Margrethe Kruse, ICN President 1969 to 1973. From AJN Collection.*

position. She convinced the board to delay hiring until Herwitz could be persuaded to add her name to the pool of applicants: "It is not two months since she came to a highly complicated office, and in that short time she has been able to acquaint herself with the work at headquarters and win the confidence of both the professional and general staff members. It is not too much to say that she has started to introduce a sense of stability and a happier atmosphere at Headquarters. There is no doubt that she is extremely interested in ICN and its affairs and with a little more time it may well be that she will be interested in applying for the post."[5]

After some persuasion, Herwitz formally applied for the position, was accepted, and appointed ICN's new executive director on October 9, 1970.[6] A graduate of Beth Israel School of Nursing in Boston, Massachusetts, Herwitz had prior administrative experience as the director of the American Nurses Association Economic Security Program (1952–1964) and associate executive director for Programs (1964–1970). Receiving both baccalaureate and master's degrees from Teachers College, Columbia University in New York City, she later served as a captain in the Army Nurses Corps during World War II.[7]

With its internal operations now under control, the ICN continued its campaign to increase membership. In the year before Herwitz's hire, 11 new countries joined ICN at the 14th Quadrennial Congress in Montreal, Canada in 1969: Argentina, Bolivia, Bermuda, Costa Rica, Ecuador, Lebanon, Morocco, Nepal, Portugal, Salvador, and Uganda. Lebanon and Morocco represented the organization's first two nurse associations from predominantly Muslim countries.

Lebanon, a former French colony until its independence in 1943, patterned its nurses' training after an eclectic French, German, American, and British model. Early Lebanese nursing began in 1847 when the French Sisters of Charity developed a small hospital next to their convent. In 1860, the Prussian Knights of the Order of St. John established their hospital and staffed it with German Deaconess nurses educated at Kaiserswerth. Later, in 1905, the Syrian Protestant College founded its hospital and opened a school of nursing under the direction of Jane Van Zandt, a graduate of the New York Postgraduate Medical School and colleague of American Annie Goodrich.[8] The combined influence of Christian doctrine and Western nursing practice distinguished Lebanon from its neighbor, Morocco, with its Muslim tradition and largely male nurse workforce.

## Unity Through Communication

Agreeing with Agnes Ohlson that "one of the ways we get nursing's message across to the world is to get the message across to nurses themselves," Herwitz renewed the ICN's commitment to global communication.[9] One of the earliest examples of the organization's commitment to the globalization of nursing and health care was its formal endorsement of the United Nations Universal Declaration of Human Rights in 1971. Referred to by Herwitz as "a mirror image of why we became nurses—because we believe in the rights of man and the dignity and worth of each human being," the UN Declaration promoted international cooperation in securing worldwide human rights and peace.[10]

Implemented by the United Nations Educational, Scientific and Cultural Organization (UNESCO), the document contained, among other things, stringent clauses against "the continuing pernicious influence of colonialism, neocolonialism, racialism, fascism, and other antihumanistic concepts on the intellectual life of the peoples of a number of countries."[11] The ICN's support of the document symbolized a transition in its "imagined community." That is, by endorsing this international policy, the ICN allied itself with the international community, creating new and competing tensions between the interests of some of its member nations and international interests.

## Ungraceful Withdrawal

A good example of the ICN's difficulty holding national and international interests in equilibrium is the story of the South African Nurses Association's (SANA) 1973 withdrawal from ICN membership.[12] Three years before the ICN officially recognized the UN Declaration, the Swedish Nurses Association (SNA) revisited the issue of SANA's apartheid policies. In a series of letters to the ICN Board of Directors, the SNA demanded a review of SANA's racial classification system. Stressing her association's historical stance against racial discrimination, SNA Executive Secretary Gunvor Stjernlof demanded that SANA voluntarily withdraw from membership or be forcibly expelled.[13]

The board of directors finally confronted SANA directly. As an associate member of UNESCO, ICN was expected to comply with the provisions enshrined within UNESCO policy. John E. Fobes, UNESCO's acting director general, complained to Herwitz about SANA's racially discriminative practices and finally suspended the ICN/UNESCO alliance on the grounds that ICN included "branches, sections, affiliates or constituted parts in the Republic of South Africa, Southern Rhodesia, or Portuguese-dominated African territories."[14]

Responding to the UNESCO suspension, Herwitz wrote to SANA President P. H. Harrison. She reiterated the ICN's position on human rights and requested that SANA "provide concrete evidence of the efforts they have made to demonstrate their policy against apartheid whether the efforts have had positive or negative results."[15] In a delayed response, SANA Executive Director D. H. Radloff reminded Herwitz of her association's 50-year ICN membership and expressed disapproval of the UNESCO decision. Moreover, Radloff argued that SANA was not in violation of ICN membership requirements particularly because it "subscribed to the United Nation's Declaration of Human Rights," which together with the ICN Code of Ethics, were "incorporated in teaching all nurses their responsibilities toward their patients and the communities they serve. Suspension from UNESCO," Radloff ended, "would not in any way affect *nursing* responsibilities or the objectives of ICN."[16]

Herwitz explained the SANA situation to the board of directors as a conflict between national and international politics: "There should seem to be two issues involved. One is the external matter of ICN and public relations vis-a-vis UNESCO and the world at large. If we are in fact reinstated [to full membership] that will be good for our image. The other issue is an *internal* one between ICN and its member association in South Africa."[17] Herwitz realized that if ICN aligned with the international community against SANA, it risked losing a valuable longstanding member; if it sided with SANA, it risked isolation from the international community.

When the revised 1972 South African Nursing Act still included the 1957 stipulation that, "No person shall be appointed or elected as a member of the Council who is not a South African citizen and a white person," the ICN Board of Directors was pressed to action. SANA President Dr. Charlotte Searle was asked to explain SANA's differential treatment of white and nonwhite nurses at the 1973 Board of Directors meeting in Mexico City. She explained that, in concordance with South African law, only white nurses could serve on the SANA Board of Directors; the admission of nonwhite nurses to board positions was illegal. When asked whether SANA would be willing to elect nonwhites to the SANA Board, Searle submitted, "If we are to be involved in a political struggle to achieve that goal, the answer must be no."[18]

Although SANA was legally bound to an all-white board, Searle pointed with pride to growing trends of nonwhite nurse participation within the nurses association. Claiming that "opportunities for the professional development of nonwhite nurses and the professional benefits which have accrued to these nurses through the efforts of the Board of the SANA are superior in many respects to those which exist for nurses in many Western countries," Searle presented statistics showing rising numbers of registered professional nurses among the nonwhite Bantu and Coloured and Indian groups.[19] These trends had been reported earlier in an article published in the *American Journal of Nursing* by American nurse Barbara Beal. Beal, a nurse at Rancho Los Amigos Hospital in Downey, California, visited South African hospitals and training schools in 1969 and concluded: "Apartheid has had an unexpected effect . . . while one does find nurses of one race caring for patients of another race, the official aim here is for each race to become equipped to care for its own people . . . [since apartheid] there has been tremendous acceleration in the training of nonwhite nurses."[20]

Although the ICN Board of Directors ultimately recognized discrimination within the SANA as reflected in the composition of its board, it still did not recommend expulsion.[21] Rather, secure with the international community behind it, it urged SANA to withdraw voluntarily from membership.[22]

The South African Nurses Association quietly withdrew from ICN membership on July 21, 1973, ostensibly on grounds of finance.[23] *Nursing Times* editor Michael Bangs and others criticized SANA's "ungraceful withdrawal."[24] SANA member A. F. S. Towert was furious that the SANA Board made a decision to withdraw from ICN membership without first consulting its constituency. Towert refused to accept "Miss Harrison's rationalising" especially because there was "no mention made that South Africa had been given until 1975 to 'put her house in order.'"[25] "That withdrawal was preferable to expulsion is acceptable," Towert conceded, "but please let us see it for what it was, a face-saving device necessitated by our present discriminatory laws."[26]

SANA's withdrawal marked ICN's closer identification with the international community and redefinition of its international identity. Its endorsement of UNESCO policy signified ICN's growing confidence as nursing's global voice with all of its implicit opportunity and responsibility.[27]

## Expanding Nursing's Voice

By the 1970s, "professional responsibility" became a familiar refrain in advertising nurses' role in international health care policy and practice. Formalized in the proclamation of an International Nurses Day coinciding with Florence Nightingale's May 12th birthday, ICN began developing theme-based educational materials for distribution to member associations. The first theme "Unity" attempted to create "a concerted, world wide impact on one health problem." In 1972, the Nurses Day theme, "The Nurse's Role in Policy-making and Planning," invited nurses to participate in local, national, and international health planning and policy making. The following year, "The Nurse's Role in Safeguarding the Environment" emphasized nurses' responsibility for public hygiene and sanitation.

The ICN's first public health stance was its endorsement of the World Health Organization's report on the "Limitation of Smoking." ICN leaders and platform speakers at the May 1973 Council of National Representatives meeting in Mexico City abstained from smoking to set an example for others.[28] Smoking restrictions were not enforced among the general nursing audience.[29]

A year later, the ICN lobbied the 48-man governing body of the International Labour Office (ILO) to place the "Report on Conditions of Work and Life of Nursing Personnel" on the 1976 ILO Labour Conference agenda.[30] The report, compiled by a committee of ILO and WHO representatives chaired by Royal Australian Nursing Federation member Mary Patten, aimed to create universal standards for nurses' socioeconomic welfare. Initially reviewed by the 24-physician WHO Executive Board and rejected as "infelicitous" and "impertinent," the report was then sent to the ILO Governing Board for a final decision. The ILO Board's 48 members included 12 representatives from the worker's side, 12 employer delegates, and 24 government officials.

Given the board's heavy state-represented composition, the ICN encouraged its 74 member associations to contact their local government representatives as a means to influence the decision outcome. ICN leaders made personal contact with WHO/ILO Committee experts and "talked [themselves] hoarse" to gather necessary support. When the ILO Board reconvened on May 31, 1974, the ICN's lobbying efforts proved successful; the report was passed unanimously. Herwitz wrote enthusiastically to the ICN Board of Directors: "And we won! Nobody thought we would but we did. The worker's side votes went for our item, the employers' side 12 votes were solid 'for the nurses' and about 11 governments also supported putting the item on the 1976 Labour Conference agenda . . . they were all surprised themselves to see what strong support we had."[31]

In the wake of the ICN's victorious campaign, Herwitz pressed further for improved internal communication. She initiated a monthly newsletter along with quarterly financial statements to the board of directors to keep it appraised of ICN's numerous activities and up-to-the-moment financial status. She also maintained weekly correspondence with Kruse and her successor, Dorothy Cornelius. The *International Nursing Review* (*INR*) was reformatted and began soliciting manuscripts from all member associations. Educational pamphlets were distributed world-wide to spread ICN's agenda and promote the organization's appeal to potential new members.

Research was encouraged as a means to articulate nursing practice and education. A $6,000 donation by the Minnesota Mining and Manufacturing Company (3M) permitted ICN to distribute Fellowship Awards to nurses seeking postgraduate study. Member associations were invited to nominate one member annually for the award. The first 3M Fellowship

---

 **ICN/3M AWARD WINNERS**

From 1970 to 1994, the ICN/3M Scholarship Program awarded grants for higher education in nursing. The 58 winners are:

|  |  |
|------|--------|
| 1970 | Berenice King of New Zealand |
| 1971 | Junko Kondo of Japan |
| 1972 | Margaret Dean of India |
| 1973 | Alice Baumgart of Canada |
| 1974 | Irma Sandoval of Costa Rica |
| 1975 | Audun Tommeras of Norway and Ibrahima Lo of Senegal |
| 1976 | Panun Boon-Long of Thailand and Poolast Jadunundun of Mauritius |
| 1977 | Hartja Kalkas of Finland and Jean Grayson of Trinidad |
| 1978 | Teresa Chopoorian of the United States and Pauline Mella of Tanzania |
| 1979 | Kola Oyedepo of Nigeria and Gnana Jayaratne of Sri Lanka |
| 1980 | Maria Rovers Zinck of Canada and Valerie Hardware of Jamaica |
| 1981 | Magda C. Vera Llamanzarea of the Philippines and Eleonore Grant Collymore of St. Lucia |
| 1982 | Carolyn Pepler of Canada, Dotnie Elaine Smith of Jamaica, and Ada Ramona Agasco of Argentina |
| 1983 | Sung-Sill Kim of Korea, Kelesitse Ttale of Botswana, and Audrey Yoke Lin Tang of Singapore |
| 1984 | Chi-Hui Lo of Taiwan, Cynthia Cecilia of Sierra Leone, and Nilda Ledezma de Gutierrez of Bolivia |
| 1985 | Urzula Krzyzanowska-Lagowska of Poland, Geraldine McCarthy of Ireland, and Ana Taukapa Fotu of Tonga |
| 1986 | Judith Martha Clift of Austria, Blanca H. Roa Ghiselini of Chile, and Kgomotso Kenaope Badimela of Botswana |
| 1987 | Pailin Nukulkij of Thailand, Sharon McKinley of Australia, and Maroulla Antoniou of Cyprus |

*(continued)*

| ICN/3M AWARD WINNERS (CONTINUED) |
|---|
| 1988 | Puangtip Chaiphibalsarisdi of Thailand, Merian Litchfield Campbell of New Zealand, and Wilberforce Adade of Ghana |
| 1989 | Gloria Ortiz Blanco of Puerto Rico, Tamar Ben-Or of Israel, and Despina Sapountzi of Greece |
| 1990 | Andreas Paviakis of Cyprus, Speciosa Mbabali of Uganda, and Kumbalatra Wljlnayake of Sri Lanka |
| 1991 | Mary Ama Opare of Ghana, Nurith Wagner of Israel, and Donna R. Hodnicki of the United States |
| 1992 | Hazel Margaret Mackenzie of the United Kingdom, Faustina Oware-Gyekye of Ghana, and Lyman Albian R. Phillips of Barbados |
| 1993 | Frank Lamendola of the United States, Mirit Shiloa of Israel, and Dorcas S. Phiri of Zambia |
| 1994 | Monica Bruce of Trinidad and Tobago, Maria Gundmundsdottir of Iceland, and Surandra Beebakhy of Mauritius |

Award was awarded to New Zealand's Berenice King in 1970. Japan's Junko Kondo followed in 1971, with India's Margaret Dean and Canada's Alice Baumgart in 1972 and 1973, respectively. In 1975, the 3M Award was doubled to allow for the dispensation of two annual awards in post-basic training and graduate study. Thailand's Panun Boon-Long and Mauritius' Poolast Jadunundun were selected from 47 applicants in 1976; Hartja Kalkas of Finland and Jean Grayson from Trinidad and Tobago from a pool of 44 the following year.[32]

Elected president at the 1973 Quadrennial Congress in Mexico City under the watchword "flexibility," American Dorothy Cornelius outlined three major objectives for the years ahead: increase ICN membership; elicit and utilize input from individual members of national associations; and strengthen communication between the ICN Board of Directors and member associations.[33] An ICN Board member from 1969 to 1973, ANA president from 1968 to 1970 and president of the American Journal of Nursing Company from 1967 to 1968, Cornelius was familiar with the more practical aspects of organizational leadership. Reflecting on the ICN's past and future, Cornelius argued that if ICN aimed to survive in the years ahead, it would need to "bend without breaking."[34]

Cornelius' first objective, to increase ICN membership, stemmed from the twin problem of ICN's ongoing financial difficulties and its heavy dependence on membership dues. Increased spending without a requisite increase in membership or membership dues had created an enormous

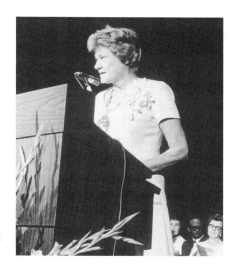

**FIGURE 5-2**
*Dorothy Cornelius, ICN President
1973 to 1977. From AJN Collection.*

budget deficit; the 1974–1975 budget report showed expenditures of Swiss Francs (SF) 134,940 over income.[35]

Kruse criticized her own quadrennium as a time when ICN was "ambitious beyond [its] resources and did not succeed in bringing means and ends into balance."[36] Agreeing with Kruse in a summary of her first years in office, Cornelius noted, "The realism of the financial picture of ICN has often sent us down another path . . . .I believe that ICN has stretched its resources nearly to the point when the elasticity we have grown accustomed to must be questioned."[37]

The ICN's deteriorating financial picture forced a reexamination of membership criteria. Although the total number of national nurses associations (NNAs) had increased gradually over the previous quadrennium, individual membership within the 74 member countries had declined 4.6% between 1969 and 1973, from 543,458 to 518,285 members.[38] Because annual dues were paid on a per capita basis, the loss of individual members had deleterious consequences on ICN's budget.

Kruse correlated declining numbers with ICN's stringent "nurses only" criteria that excluded certain types of nurses from association membership without consideration of the cultural variations in nurses' work. She argued for more localized control of membership through the nursing associations: "The ICN is the international spokesman for nursing and nurses, but it is not a supranational body . . . it must be left to the countries to decide their own patterns of nursing and to the associations to decide their own patterns of organization, including their criteria for membership."[39]

Advocating a national interpretation of nurse membership over an international one, Kruse challenged Fenwick's notion of the universality of nurses' work. As Kruse put it, "The work of nurses varies from one country to another according to the needs of the people and the financial and human resources of the country."[40] The path to "real unity" among nurses worldwide, she insisted, was acknowledgment of the differences between cultures and associations rather than the assumption and encouragement of cultural and professional hegemony. Kruse's view ultimately influenced ICN's redefinition of "nurse" to include both first-level and second-level nurses.

The "first-level nurse," coined by the Professional Services Committee at the 1973 CNR meeting, was broadly defined as "a person who has completed a programme of basic nursing education and is qualified and authorized in her/his country to provide responsible and competent professional service for the promotion of health, the prevention of illness, the care of the sick, and rehabilitation."[41] Basic nursing education was interpreted as "a planned educational programme which provides a broad and sound foundation for the effective practice of professional nursing and a basis for post-basic education."[42] A generalist in training and practice, the first-level nurse was distinguished from the more specialized second-level or auxiliary nurse, which included enrolled nurses, practical nurses, assistant nurses, and specialist nurses in the care of children and community.

Previously rejected for membership at the Fourteenth Quadrennial Congress in Montreal in 1969, second-level nurses were reconsidered after results from a membership survey revealed the number, education, role, and status of various levels of auxiliary nursing personnel throughout the world.[43] Of the 40 associations who answered the questionnaire, only Japan admitted assistant nurses as full association members. Indeed, most (94,412) of Japan's reported membership (131,912) in 1973 were second-level nursing personnel.[44] Although Japan's 1948 Public Health Nurse, Midwife, and Nurse Law differentiated levels of nurses and raised nursing education to a professional level, distinction between types and levels of nurses remained unclear. Registered nurses were defined as "females li-

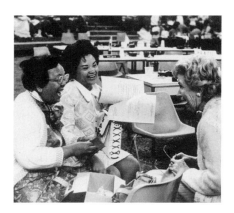

FIGURE 5-3
*Delegates happy to be at the 1973 ICN Congress in Mexico. From AJN Collection.*

censed by the Minister for Health and Welfare who practice nursing for the injured sick or women in childbirth or assist medical examination and treatment"; assistant nurses were "females practicing the practices of nurses under the direction of a medical practitioner, dentist, or registered nurse."[45] Although a 1968 revised law concerning public health nurses (*Hokenfus*), midwives (*Sanbas*, now called *Josanpus*), and registered nurses aimed to distinguish nurses by practice and educational characteristics, there was often no work differentiation between assistant nurses and professional nurses.[46]

Most of the other queried member associations, even those who relied heavily on auxiliary nursing personnel, agreed that auxiliary nurses should form their own associations or be given associate membership within national associations.[47] Although nearly reaching consensus, any board decision to admit second-level nurses to membership was deferred until 1975.

In 1973, the CNR supported a motion to increase dues payments for first level nurses from SF 1.60 to 2.50 (US $0.52 to $0.85). Although dues had remained unchanged for 12 years, most of the national representatives voted against the proposed increase. Representatives from Sierra Leone and Chile, for example, argued that a dues increase would strain their already struggling associations. South Africa called the dues proposal "unjustifiable," claiming that raising dues impeded expansion efforts by many national associations.[48] Identifying its own financial difficulties, the Kenyan association supported a moderate increase to SF 2.0, a motion that was soundly defeated.[49]

On January 1, 1976, the ICN's 84 member associations finally approved a dues increase to SF 2.20 for first-level nurses and, approving membership for auxiliary nurses, SF 1.10 for second-level nurses. Because many countries expressed difficulty or inability to pay the new rates, however, the Council of National Representatives reviewed six sliding scale proposals that considered associations' size and ability to pay. It was noted that 66 of the 84 member associations had fewer than 5,000 members, 10 had between 5,000 and 15,000, and the remaining 8 had over 15,000 member nurses. The United States, Canada, and Japan stood apart among the eight larger associations with memberships greater than 100,000.[50]

Given the per capita formula, great care was exercised to determine who could pay, who could not, and at what rate members who could pay were assigned. Lowering dues rates for poorer countries with fewer members, for example, reduced the ICN's overall income and had the potential to foster resentment among the larger dues-paying nations. The ICN was particularly concerned that larger nations would withdraw from membership because, despite their greater financial obligation, they did not benefit through greater organizational representation. All nations, small or large, rich or poor, were equally represented at the Council of National Representatives.

## The Imagined Community in New Territories

Although increasing membership was linked to the ICN's financial solvency, it also fulfilled the organization's goal of globalizing nursing. The inclusion of the Bahamas, Senegal, Tanzania, Sudan, Nicaragua, and Zaire in 1973; Fiji, Swaziland, Mauritius, St. Lucia, and Puerto Rico in 1975; and Paraguay and Western Samoa in 1977 spread nursing's "message" into more exotic areas around the globe.[51] Cornelius viewed this "penetration of new territories" as critical to ICN's survival and influence especially because the ICN's growth coincided with the declining success of other international organizations. "I think we have a right to be proud of this growth," Herwitz wrote in a circular letter to the board of directors in December 1976, "particularly at a time when our medical colleagues seem to be moving in the opposite direction . . . an article in the paper reported that the medical associations of Canada, Switzerland, and Austria were withdrawing from the World Medical Association."[52]

Although the ICN exhibited unparalleled growth among professional health organizations, not all of its efforts to "penetrate new territories" were successful. Adele Herwitz's 1975 visit to Russia, sponsored by the Medical Workers Union, yielded limited information about the status of the Russian Nurses' Organization.[53] Herwitz's visit followed years of futile efforts to associate with the Russian nurses. As described earlier by Kruse, " . . . we have tried, through the Health Workers Union of the USSR to

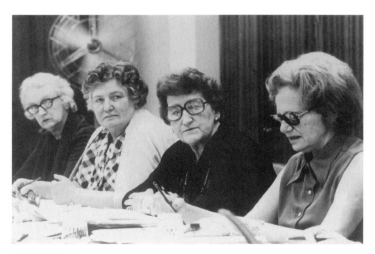

**FIGURE 5-4**
*At an ICN Board of Directors Meeting, 1974. From left: Hildegard Peplau (USA), Olive Anstey, who would become ICN President (1977 to 1981), Ingrid Hamelin (Finland) and Hamuda Mar-Haim (Israel). From ICN Collection.*

get in touch with the nurses in the USSR . . . so far, no results have been obtained."[54] Despite a long history of unsuccessful attempts to affiliate with Russian nurses, the ICN's regular and often persistent contact with other countries proved invaluable to its growing international influence.

When the Council of National Representatives met in Singapore in 1975, it represented the first meeting of ICN in a Southeast Asian country. Cornelius commented on the importance of this meeting to the ICN's external image: "As ICN becomes increasingly the spokesman for nursing worldwide and as our relationship with other organizations and groups grows, it is fitting that we should be meeting here in this part of the world. It is by reminding ourselves of our truly international character and make-up that we are able to put into proper perspective the small day-to-day problems that we face and solve."[55]

But while the ICN expanded its community as a means to wider global influence, the Royal College of Nursing and National Council of Nurses of the United Kingdom (RCN) issued a surprise decree. Claiming that it disagreed with the ICN's direction for change and unwilling to support "the substantial and increasing financial commitment involved in contin-ued membership," the RCN threatened to withdraw from membership by December 31, 1975.[56] In the RCN's view, the ICN's expansionist agenda was more flexible than its budget and "adopted a totally unrealistic posi-tion that insisted on a continuing wide-ranging role for the ICN while withholding the financial means to fulfill this role."[57]

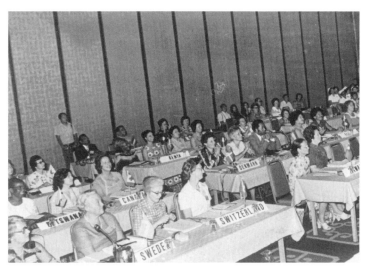

**FIGURE 5-5**
*Council of National Representatives, 1975, Singapore. From AJN Collection.*

Writing of this to the board, Herwitz noted that the RCN dictum was generated by only 2% of its membership. "It is now obvious that the issue of withdrawing from ICN was not the result of pressure on the leadership from the membership but rather the idea of a selected few among the leadership . . . the fact that 495 voted for withdrawing from ICN and 301 voted to stay in ICN means that 194 people decided for 42,000. We are saddened by the news and do honestly believe that nursing in the U.K. will be weakened by this self-imposed isolation."[58]

Cornelius viewed the RCN's imminent disassociation more broadly as a loss to international nursing: "While the RCN membership is less than 7% of the total ICN membership, the loss is regrettable . . . members of the RCN lose their voice in international affairs and ICN loses future leadership from the RCN."[59]

The RCN's decision to withdraw from ICN membership coincided with Great Britain's growing inflation and the declining value of the English pound against the Swiss franc. Centering its complaints on financial concerns, the RCN nonetheless freely expressed its criticism of the ICN's role in international nursing, its forward agenda, its shifting location from London to Geneva, and a host of other issues.[60] Rumors held that the RCN's threat of withdrawal had less to do with the association's financial state and more to do with personal and political agendas.[61]

In the end, the RCN threat of withdrawal did not materialize. The association remained in ICN membership after a revote at the RCN Annual General Meeting on November 26, 1975 reversed the April decision by a three-to-one margin.[62] Although the true motive behind the RCN's threat of withdrawal can only be speculated, the RCN story is emblematic of the importance of money and politics in nursing education, practice, and policy. Certainly, uncertain economies played a central role in transforming nursing around the world in the 1970s.

As many countries experienced economic strain, nurses, facing unemployment or inadequate remuneration in their own countries, migrated to nations claiming critical nurse shortages. The massive exodus of nursing and other health care personnel prompted the World Health Organization (WHO) to sponsor a study analyzing its health policy implications. Authors Alfonso Mejia, Helena Pizurki, and Erica Royston noted a dearth of data on nurses with which to forge a comprehensive or meaningful analysis.[63] Nonetheless, many nurses associations complained of the "brain drain" of nursing personnel from their countries to the United States, Canada, and others.[64]

## A Legacy of Fortune and Scholarship

In 1975, at the height of the ICN's financial worries, former Executive Secretary Christiane Reimann offered ICN a two-part gift of "fortune and property." In two wills written in 1968, Reimann provided income from her Danish investments for an annual award (around $6,000) to "a nurse who has made a significant contribution to nursing for the benefit of mankind or the nursing profession" and her $300,000 Sicilian Villa Fegotto for use as a nurses' vacation spot or rest home.[65]

Seven years later, fearing a Communist rise to power in Italy, Reimann offered to transfer her property to the ICN with the stipulation that she remain there until her death. Although on its face a generous gesture, Reimann's bequest did not include maintenance costs that ICN would necessarily incur once the property transferred ownership. Nor did it factor in the costly round-the-clock personal assistance Reimann would require.

Visiting Reimann at her estate in 1975 to discuss the proposed transfer of property, Herwitz returned to Geneva "like a piece of driftwood washed up on the beach after a bad storm!"[66] Reimann, now nearly blind and deaf, had fallen the night before Herwitz's visit. Disoriented after her fall, the 88-year-old Reimann reverted to Danish or Italian such that discussion about the property matter was impossible.

A few months later, Cornelius, Kruse and Herwitz agreed to revisit Reimann as a "delegation," particularly after Reimann still refused to establish an adjoining foundation for property maintenance costs. The visit was canceled, however, when Cornelius became ill. Herwitz maintained written correspondence with Reimann until, exasperated, she wrote to the board, "Perhaps it sounds ungrateful but I know you will understand if I say the whole subject is taking more time and energy than one would expect to devote to 'a gift.' I told our lawyer the matter was taking on the overtones of a bad Italian opera except that I don't know how to sing and can't seem to get off the stage."[67]

Ultimately, Reimann donated her property to the University of Syracusa in 1977. Money was set aside for the coveted Hygieia Prize, or Christiane Reimann Award, upon Reimann's death in 1979. Issued every 4 years, the first award was given to Virginia Henderson in 1985 for her world-renowned work "Basic Principles of Nursing Care."

## Accounts and Accountability

In 1977, Herwitz resigned as ICN executive director and returned to the United States to become the first executive director of the newly created Commission on Graduates of Foreign Nursing Schools (CGFNS). British nurse Barbara Fawkes took over as executive director until Scotland's Winifred Logan replaced her in April 1978, a position she held until a car accident in Nairobi forced her early retirement in August 1980. Nurse advisor Doris Krebs then served as acting executive director until Constance Holleran's appointment in 1981.

Dorothy Cornelius pronounced the watchword "accountability" for newly elected President Olive E. Anstey's quadrennium (1977–1981). Anstey, past president of the Royal Australian Nursing Federation and member of the board of directors, had previously practiced as a public health nurse, ward sister at the Royal Prince Alfred Hospital, and sister-in-charge of operating theaters and staff nurse at the Royal Perth Hospital. Israel's Rebecca Bergman was elected first vice president, Canadian Verna Huffman Splane second vice president, and American Hildegard Peplau third vice president.

Cornelius' choice of "accountability" was prompted by her belief that "those who work together in ICN for organized nursing must demonstrate a two-fold accountability—as individual practitioners and as members of the association who formulate policy for ICN."[68] Accountability denied "isolationism in nursing" and embraced the philosophy of "spreading nursing's knowledge and caring to the most remote areas of the world."[69]

In step with Cornelius' thinking, Anstey prioritized improvement of nurses' global socioeconomic welfare. The *Socio-Economic News* kept its readers appraised of news and information pertaining to the ICN's work in this area.[70] Discussions of labor relations, collective bargaining and unionization, practice liability, remuneration, working conditions, professional practice, and "comparable worth" filled its pages. The ICN publication *What About Me? Caring for the Carers*, edited by Sheila Quinn, elaborated on the socioeconomic welfare of nurses as ICN's "top priority."[71]

Anstey's second objective, to increase nursing's role in primary care, followed the 1977 adoption of the Health for All by the Year 2000 program by the World Health Assembly. With substantial evidence that most of

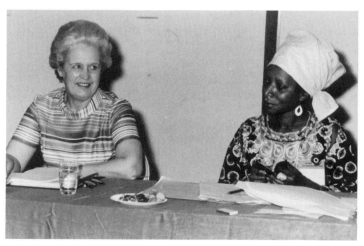

**FIGURE 5-6**
*Sheila Quinn, ICN Executive 1968 to 1970 and Eunice Muringo Kiereini, later ICN President, attending the ICN Congress in Tokyo, in 1977. From AJN Collection.*

the world's population was in poor health and over 70% of the population in developing nations had no access to health care services whatsoever, Health for All aimed for universal health care access.

In 1978, primary care was identified as the vehicle for attaining health for all at the WHO/UNICEF-sponsored International Conference of Primary Health Care in Alma Ata, USSR. Defining primary health care as "essential health care," the Alma Ata Declaration called for all national governments to formulate national policies, strategies, and plans of action to ensure accessible, cost-effective health services for individuals and families.[72] Jamaican nurse and board member Syringa Marshall-Barnett, Executive Director Winifred Logan, and nurse advisor Doris Krebs represented ICN at the conference. A year later, they committed ICN to "making primary care an effective reality" in their coauthored publication "Contribution of Nursing to Primary Health Care."[73]

Following through on its commitment, the ICN held its "Symposium on Nursing in Primary Health Care" at the 1981 Congress in Los Angeles, California. Proposing strategies for local action by member associations and international influence by ICN, efforts were made to strengthen and prescribe nurses' roles and contributions in the delivery of primary health care over the next decade.[74]

One of the ICN's first primary health care stances was its endorsement of the WHO/UNICEF position against female excision, circumcision, and mutilation. The ICN's sanction, proposed by the Royal Australian Nursing Federation, called for the abolition of female circumcision on grounds of its health danger and "cost" in human lives, hospitalization, and lost work time.[75] A background document presented at the 1981 board of directors meeting in Los Angeles detailed the specific types of female genital mutilation: circumcision (sunna), excision/clitoridectomy, and infibulation/pharaonic circumcision, and the health risks associated with each procedure.

The ICN's position against female genital mutilation coincided with UNICEF's International Year of the Child campaign and followed the first international meeting on female circumcision: the WHO Regional Seminar in Traditional Practices Affecting the Health of Women in Khartoum, Sudan. At that meeting, recommendations were made for clearly defined national policies aimed at abolishing genital mutilation of girls and women. Keynote speaker, Fran P. Hosken, special advisor to WHO and the editor of *Women's International Network News* (WIN), shared the findings of her 6-year study of genital mutilation in Africa. Concluding that "these 2000 year old genital operations are rapidly spreading due to population growth and to a conspiracy of silence by all international development agencies working in Africa," Hosken challenged international agencies to intervene in a practice with immediate and long-term physical and psychological consequences for women and children. Hosken, who published three editions of *The Hosken Report: Genital and Sexual Mutilation of Females*, estimated that 74 million girls (usually between the ages of 5 and 8) and women were victims of "sexual castration" justified by "tradition."[76]

ICN support for specific public health care issues demonstrated the organization's growing accountability in matters of international concern. Other specific endorsements related to nursing education, such as the American Nurses Association's proposal to include mental health content in undergraduate nursing curriculums can also be seen as more broadly related to the public's health.[77]

## Growth on Many Levels

In 1981, newly appointed Executive Director Constance Holleran outlined her objectives for the 1980s: strengthen member nursing associations, promote the economic well-being of nurses, foster the efforts of nursing in primary care, continue international relations, and maintain active publication.

Holleran earned a nursing diploma at Massachusetts General Hospital, Boston, Massachusetts in 1956, a BSN in 1958 from Teachers College, Columbia University, New York and an MSN in Nursing Education Administration from Catholic University of America, Washington, DC, in 1965. Between 1965 and 1970, she served as nurse consultant and project grants section chief with the Division of Nursing, United States Public Health Service, Department of Health, Education, and Welfare. From 1971 until her ICN executive director appointment in March 1981, Hol-

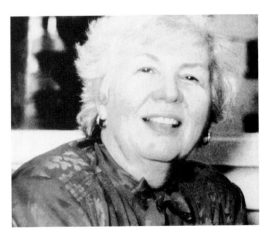

**FIGURE 5-7**
*Constance Holleran, ICN Executive Director, 1981 to 1996. From AJN Collection.*

leran was deputy executive director for Government Relations for the ANA in Washington, DC.[78]

Holleran's five-part agenda reflected both the organization's longstanding efforts to establish itself as nursing's international voice as well as her own personal agenda for change. Although she would later recall that her first year in office was "very easy, very nice," one of Holleran's earliest concerns was ICN's precarious financial status.[79] Holleran encouraged the board of directors to seek outside funding rather than continue dependence on membership dues and to prioritize activities until the budget could be stabilized: ". . . we cannot afford to dilute our efforts with many other activities we might like to do but that are not in our own priorities . . . it seems better to do a few things at a time and do them well."[80]

The 17th Quadrennial Congress in Los Angeles, California (1981), "Health Care for All—Challenge for Nursing," committed ICN further to helping individuals attain healthy productive lives.[81] Olive Anstey handed down the watchword "freedom" to newly elected President Eunice Muringo Kiereini, who ran unopposed to become the first African nurse elected to ICN's highest executive position.[82] Former Chief Nursing Officer of the Ministry of Health in Nairobi and Kenya, Kiereini was also the founding member and former chairperson of the National Nurses' Association of Kenya. A graduate of Southampton General Hospital, Southampton, England, Kiereini later studied at Simpson Maternity Hospital in Edinburgh, Scotland toward midwife certification.

Kiereini's nomination corresponded with the impressive slate of African states admitted to ICN membership in the early 1980s: Tonga and Seychelles in 1980, Malawi and Lesotho in 1981, and Zimbabwe and Burkina Faso in 1983. It also coincided with a world still struggling with

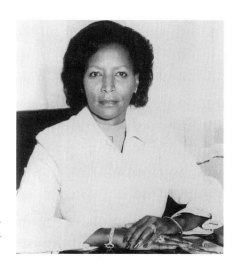

**FIGURE 5-8**
*Eunice Muringo Kiereini, ICN President 1981 to 1985. From ICN Collection.*

associated pressing issues for nurses. The Socioeconomic Welfare Program (SEW), first developed and active between 1961 and 1966 and then phased out, was resuscitated in an attempt to address nurses' welfare in the workplace. The committee's first newsletter, printed in February 1980, identified ways in which member associations could help each other and themselves.[83] Other SEW publications, such as the "Caring for the Carers" series, addressed important workplace issues such as collective bargaining, rights negotiation, and dispute settlement.[84]

Unstable employment of nurses once again threatened the stability of many national associations and their ability to raise dues. In 1983, a new system tied dues to annual World Bank GNP data, thus giving consideration to the financial hardships of many national associations created by currency restrictions, inflation, and devaluation of money. By the early 1980s, Holleran happily reported ICN's "comfortable financial situation," which she attributed to careful management and closely watched investments. ICN also successfully obtained outside funding for several key projects such as the Primary Health Care (PHC) workshop series (funded by Canada [CIDA], Norway [NORAD], UNICEF, and PAHO), the Care of the Aging monograph (funded by WHO), and the SEW workshop in Nairobi (funded through Denmark's DANIDA).[85] Holleran noted later that fundraising, likened to and rejected as "political involvement" in earlier years, moved ICN into a more corporate (business) model of organization over its previous status as a developing agency.[86]

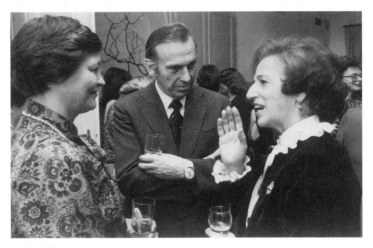

**FIGURE 5-9**
*Kirsten Stallknecht (Denmark), Halfdan Mahler (General Director, WHO), and Helen Mussallem (Canada) at ICN gathering, 1982. From ICN Collection.*

| Growth Rates of ICN Membership Countries With Largest Memberships | | | | |
|---|---|---|---|---|
| Country | 1980 | 1985 | Growth (%) | Percentage of ICN (%) |
| Japan | 157,111 | 157,300 | 0.12 | 15.0 |
| USA | 156,712 | 165,656 | 5.7 | 16.0 |
| Canada | 127,312 | 175,402 | 37.8 | 17.0 |
| UK | 99,387 | 168,704 | 69.7 | 16.0 |
| Sweden | 51,564 | 61,809 | 19.9 | 6.0 |
| Denmark | 35,395 | 40,722 | 15.0 | 4.0 |
| Australia | 30,670 | 33,847 | 10.4 | 3.0 |
| Norway | 24,416 | 32,020 | 31.1 | 3.0 |
| Spain | 25,000 | 25,000 | — | 2.0 |
| Finland | 22,417 | 24,707 | 10.2 | 2.0 |
| Switzerland | 12,099 | 12,134 | 0.29 | 1.0 |

ICN membership grew 18% between 1980 and 1985, from 862,123 to 1,056,066 members. Increased membership translated into increased dues payments and revenue. Of the 97 countries in association by 1985, 11—Japan, United States, Canada, UK, Sweden, Denmark, Australia, Spain, Norway, Finland, and Switzerland—represented 86% of ICN members.[87] Four associations exceeded memberships of 100,000, 1 had member-

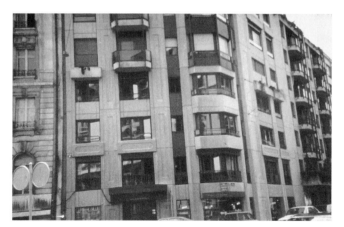

**FIGURE 5-10**
*ICN Headquarters at 3, Place Jean-Marteau, Geneva, Switzerland. From Lynaugh Collection, Bryn Mawr, PA.*

ship between 50,000 and 100,000, 4 had between 25,000 and 49,999 members, 33 claimed 1,000 to 24,999, and 55 had less than 1,000 members. The countries with the smallest memberships were in Africa, South or Central America, and Southeast Asia.

As the organization increased its membership, it continued to forge working relationships with other international organizations. For example, ICN and the League of Red Cross and Red Crescent Societies (RCRCS) collaborated in the preparation of a teaching kit on human rights and the Geneva Convention. With continued success in working with the RCRCS, WHO, UNICEF, and the ILO, ICN made its headquarters in Geneva more permanent. On July 12, 1983, the ICN purchased space for its new headquarters.

## Nurses as a Social Force

When Colombian Nelly Garzon assumed her presidential duties at the ICN Congress in Tel Aviv, Israel in 1985, she was guided by the theme, "Nurses as a Social Force." Breaking tradition, Garzon named "justice" her own quadrennium watchword, to be translated "into actions that will contribute to the well-being of the people whom we serve and ourselves as members of the Nursing Profession and into the respect, defense, and promotion of human rights."[88] Justice as action, Garzon noted, would be evident in agendas prioritized during her quadrennium: the socioeconomic well-being of nurses, leadership in primary health care, development of health and nursing care policies, definition of standards of quality nursing care and education, nursing research, nursing role and function clarifica-

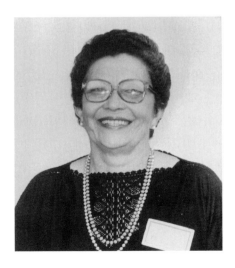

**FIGURE 5-11**
*Nelly Garzon, ICN President 1985 to 1989. From AJN Collection.*

|  CHRISTIANE REIMANN PRIZE AWARDS FROM 1985 TO 1997 | |
| --- | --- |
| 1985 | Virginia Henderson of the United States |
| 1989 | Dame Nita Barrow of Barbados |
| 1993 | Dame Sheila Quinn of the United Kingdom |
| 1997 | Mo-Im Kim of Korea and Hildegard Peplau of the United States |

tion, strengthening of nursing practice with a code of ethics, regulations to ensure the quality of nursing practice, and legal protection of nurses.[89]

Keynote speaker Hugette Labelle, deputy clerk to the Privy Council, associate secretary to the Canadian Cabinet, and former Canadian Nurses' Association president (1974–1976) examined nurses' role as social change agents more broadly. Noting that "[nurses] are intimately and inescapably tied to promoting the public good," Labelle labeled nursing's role in social change as "a goal of the greatest significance when priorities are being ordered."[90] Labelle's appeal to nurses' humanity was echoed by Israel President Chaim Herzog and outgoing ICN President Kiereini, who both implored nurses to use their knowledge to attack world problems beyond traditional health issues.

One of the "world problems" considered by the ICN was the issue of nuclear war. At the 1985 meeting of the Council of National Representatives (CNR) in Tel Aviv, delegates of the Royal Australian Nursing Federation proposed that the ICN take an active position against nuclear testing, waste dumping, and arms control.[91] Because it feared the proposal was "getting into more particularly political aspects of the issue," the CNR did not move on the resolution until 1987.[92] In June 1987, Holleran reported to the ICN Board on the Health Workers' Declaration on the Arms Race and the Threat of Nuclear War at the Moscow World Conference of Health Workers on Social Well-Being, Health, and Peace.[93]

A second health problem of worldwide concern was the growing prevalence of autoimmune deficiency syndrome (AIDS). The ICN was the first international health professional group to address the care of patients afflicted with the human immunodeficiency virus (HIV).[94] In the May/June 1985 issue of *International Nursing Review,* authors Richard Wells and Peggy Nutall urged nurses to lend their services and sympathies to combat a disease that in North America and Europe was then afflicting primarily homosexual men. "The lifestyle of many AIDS patients may be both alien and unfamiliar to some of his carers; but just as nurses cannot chose their patients, neither can patients choose their nurses."[95]

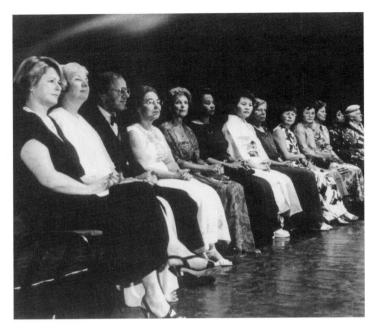

**FIGURE 5-12**
*New ICN Board at 1985 Congress in Tel Aviv, Israel. From AJN Collection.*

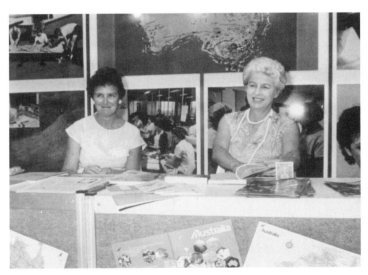

**FIGURE 5-13**
*Australian members at their booth at 1985 ICN Congress in Tel Aviv, Israel. From AJN Collection.*

The ICN's stance on HIV/AIDS signified a move away from policy statements to policy actions. Rather than simply endorsing WHO guidelines around the care of individuals with HIV/AIDS, ICN assumed an independent and active position that laid out specific nursing guidelines for persons with HIV/AIDS.

## Politics and Positions

The ICN maintained a neutral posture in member associations' internal concerns while serving as a sympathetic sounding board. During the Iran/Iraq war in the mid-1980s, for example, an Iranian nurse reported to Holleran, " . . . the Iranian Nurses Association is in not a good situation—that is, it almost does not exist. The secretary is in prison and it would be better if her name does not appear in the list . . . ."[96] Several months later, Holleran informed the board of directors of nurse consultant Mireille Kingma's abbreviated field visit to Liberia after a military coup.

In 1986, during a proposed countrywide strike by some Australian nurses, Holleran reminded the Australian Nurses Federation that "the ICN has no authority to become involved in a member organization's affairs."[97] Many associations were supporting strikes against low wages and poor work conditions in the 1980s. Nurses in Israel struck for 3 weeks in July 1986 when wage and workplace negotiations with the Israeli government broke down.[98] Expressing similar problems around wages and work to Holleran during her February 1986 field visit, the Trained Nurses' Association of India also discussed their fears regarding the implications of nationwide strike.[99] In all instances, the ICN kept physically and professionally at arms' length from member countries' national affairs.

When ICN did become involved in a case involving Chilean nurses in 1986, the complications of such involvement became very clear. As part of ICN's campaign against human rights violations, ICN President Nelly Garzon contacted Chilian President Don Augusto Pinochet Ugarte and Minister of Health Dr. Winston Chinchon Bunting regarding the status of two incarcerated nurses. It seemed the nurses were being punished for reproaching the Chilean army about the death of three schoolteachers. After Garzon's visit to one of the imprisoned nurses in May 1987, Nurses Association of Chile (NAC) Secretary Marta Aravena Vidal reminded Garzon, "Leaders should watch only for the progress of the profession, finding solutions for the problems, and keep on the outskirts of the politics in the country."[100] NAC may well have feared reprisals from the government because of ICN's involvement.

The ICN was involved in a second incident when nurse Myriam Berg Holz and physician Petro Marin were arrested and tortured for providing health care to wounded would-be assassins of the president in 1986. Executive Director Holleran wrote to Dr. Charles Grave, executive secretary of the International Commission of Health Professionals for Health and Human Rights, expressing ICN's position that the Chilean government's actions violated the Geneva Convention. The ICN's stance against those perceived injustices in Chile indicated the often-indistinct line between national and international affairs.

## Stretching the Boundaries Further

During her first years in office, Holleran increased on-site visitation to member and nonmember NNAs to increase ICN's momentum in recruiting and maintaining members. Holleran believed more extensive fieldwork strengthened NNAs and increased their effectiveness in health policy and practice. Staff visits were "essential elements" in staff program and planning.[101]

Holleran maintained contact with several NNAs herself. A visit to Taiwan (The Nurses Association of the Republic of China or NAROC) in 1986 was the first ICN visit since Verna Splane's in 1975. Meeting with NAROC President, Mrs. Chen, Holleran discussed the prospect of the Chinese Nurses Association's (CNA) readmission to ICN membership, particularly as NAROC had threatened to withdraw if CNA was reintroduced.[102]

Holleran also worked with CNA President Madam Lin Ju-Ying and representatives from the Ministries of Foreign Affairs and Public Health.[103] Eager to include both associations in membership, ICN suggested that NAROC change its name to the Nurses Association of Taiwan

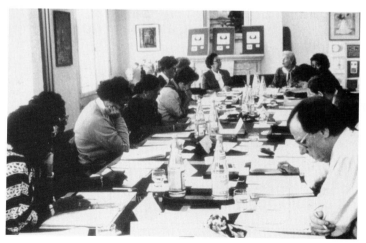

FIGURE 5-14
*ICN Board Meeting in Geneva, 1986. From ICN Collection.*

to avoid violation of the one association, one country rule. NAROC's new President, Tung-Ling Ma, although not opposed to CNA's admission, contested the name change proposal for historical reasons. As she put it:

> We would be happy to receive our mainland Chinese counterparts as fellow ICN members and to have the opportunity to meet with them in a nonpolitical environment. As nurses, we're not capitalists or communists; we're just interested in making people well. However, the Nurses Association of ROC first joined in 1922 and has always enthusiastically participated in all the activities held by ICN. We send our dues payment regularly and designate representatives to take part in CNR and the Congress. We believe that ICN is a sole professional organization where politics will not play a role, so we feel that our 68-year seniority should entitle us to at least one privilege, that of retaining our name.[104]

Ultimately, even though the CNR voted to accept CNA, it was not reintroduced to membership because its government objected to the idea of "two Chinas" represented in ICN.

Assistance to new NNAs seeking membership was also a key objective of field visitations. Mireille Kingma assessed the readiness of Cote d'Ivoire to form an NNA during her January 1988 visit. There, government-employed nurses were members of the National Union of Health Care Workers (SYNAPETESA), which made all decisions about nursing practice and policy. The nurses wished to create a section within the union that would address professional nursing issues. The Minister of Health refused to support the formation of a separate nursing association, however, and the nurses remained under government jurisdiction.[105]

The newly formed Nurses Association of Malta joined ICN shortly after Helga Morrow's visit in April 1987. Although nurses in Malta had expressed interest in joining ICN in 1978, the association finally met ICN membership criteria in 1989. Helga Morrow's visit was a first step in this successful transition.[106]

Once admitted, many smaller associations relied on ICN advisors for ongoing support. Such was the case with the newly admitted Asociacion Guatemalteca de Enfermeras Profesionales and the Asociacion Nacional de Enfermeras Salvadorenas.[107] The South African Kingdom of Lesotho's Nurses Association (LNA) experienced difficulty with organization, lack of funds, poor negotiation skills for labor conflicts, and limited space to store and maintain association files, books, and other resource materials. Visiting LNA in February 1988, Morrow recommended regular contact between ICN and the association to provide ongoing guidance and support.[108]

Site visits were also useful in assisting members to more active participation. Kingma's visit to the Association Nationale des Infirmiers et Infirmieres Diplomes d'Etat du Senegal (ANIIDES) aimed to revitalize an

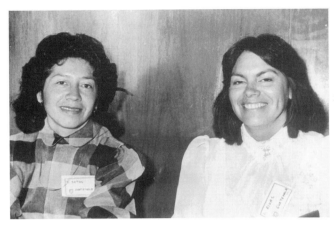

**FIGURE 5-15**
*Guatemalan delegates Lillian Rivas and Aracelly Santos at the*
*1985 ICN Congress. From AJN Collection.*

association beset with "internal conflict, personal jealousies, immigration of the NNA leadership for study abroad, decreasing finances, slander campaigns, and increasing unionism."[109] Although Kingma prepared several strategies for the association's reactivation, it withdrew from ICN membership in the early 1990s.

Late or absent dues payments, particularly from larger members, were potentially devastating to ICN's budget. As business manager Juanita C. Torres explained to the board of directors in 1988, "because one large association may find it impossible to pay their dues, we are being very careful with any expenditures."[110] At the time of her report, only SF 1.3 million of the budgeted SF 2.2 million in membership dues had been collected.

Of course, dues income varied enormously by geographic area. In 1988, 48.9% of all dues payments were from Europe, 27.1% from North America, 21.9% from Western Pacific countries, and the remaining 3.1% from associations in Africa, the Eastern Mediterranean, South and Central America, and Southeast Asia. Although Europe represented the largest percentage overall, 24 countries contributed to the total dues amount; only Canada and the United States made up North America.[111]

Of course, once dues were collected, Holleran worried how they were spent. One area of concern was the official ICN journal, *International Nursing Review*. Of the SF 2.6 million ICN income in 1987, only SF 110,000 was generated by the journal, which cost the organization SF 142,800 to produce.[112] Among the million nurse members of ICN, only 2,100 were paid subscribers, most from the United Kingdom, the United States, and Canada. Holleran was concerned that ICN was losing money

| Dues Income Received by Geographic Area—1988 | | | |
|---|---|---|---|
| Region | Number of NNAs | Dues Paid | Percentage (%) |
| Africa | 20 | 5,965 SF | 0.3 |
| Eastern Mediterranean | 8 | 11,437 SF | 0.5 |
| Europe | 24 | 1,035,399 SF | 48.9 |
| North America | 2 | 574,366 SF | 27.1 |
| South and Central America | 26 | 15,438 SF | 0.7 |
| Southeast Asia | 6 | 11,285 SF | 0.5 |
| Western Pacific | 12 | 464,277 SF | 21.9 |
| TOTAL | 98 | 2,118,168 SF | |

on an inferior product: "The purpose and goals of the *INR* have been discussed at great length in recent years. None of us are happy with it as an international journal because it does not really have the caliber articles on nursing that are of international interest and importance to nurses in all countries."[113] Improving its appeal to a broader audience became central to the journal's existence. To this end, the board approved appointment of a new editor, Nancy Vatre.

## Nurses of Tomorrow

In 1989, Mo-Im Kim became the first Asian nurse to serve as ICN president. Kim received her BS degree from the College of Nursing, Yonsei University, Korea in 1959 and her master's degree in nursing and doctorate in Public Health from Johns Hopkins University, Baltimore, Maryland. Twelve years before her election as ICN President, Kim served as president of the Korean Nurses Association and member of the Korean Parliament (1981–1985).

Kim regularly expressed her views regarding the inextricable link between life and politics. In an open letter to all 101 NNAs in membership she elaborated,

> I foresee the decade of the 1990s to be one of the most significant in history for health care systems and for the nursing profession. We are ready to meet these new challenges and ever so rapid changes and I know that many of your associations are also ready. For those of you who do not yet have clear goals, priorities and plans, I do encourage you to take time to carefully develop them. Otherwise energy and resources are squandered.[114]

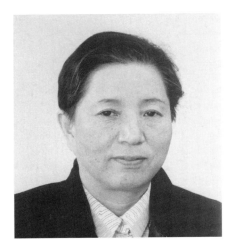

**FIGURE 5-16**
*Mo-Im Kim, ICN President 1989 to
1993. From ICN Collection.*

As Kim took office, the ICN's collective leadership also shifted toward
Asian, South American, and African representation as elected leaders
and board members from these countries, more broadly experienced and
educated than their predecessors, were prepared to take front-line positions. One emerging leader, Dame Nita Barrow of Barbados, was the 1989
recipient of the Christiane Reimann Award and keynote speaker at the
ICN's 19th Quadrennial Congress in Seoul, Korea. Dame Nita Barrow,
former ambassador to the United Nations and director of the Christian

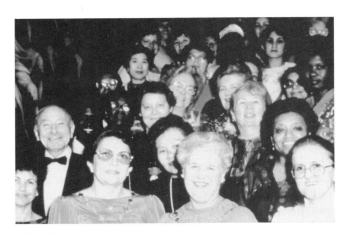

**FIGURE 5-17**
*ICN Group at the Congress in Seoul, Korea, 1989. From AJN
Collection.*

Medical Commission of the World Council of Churches (1975–1985), echoed Mo-Im Kim's call for nurses' political involvement. Linking nurses concerns to those of women more generally, Dame Nita Barrow argued, "The nurse of tomorrow will require the same skill and preparation in [politics] as her sister in other related professions in which women are in the majority, e.g. teachers. Increasing opportunities are being provided for women to acquire skill and proficiency in this area of politics. Professional concern for nursing and justice for patients should form the basis for political pressure."[115]

Dame Nita Barrow and Mo-Im Kim linked ICN's survival to its role as policy maker rather than policy follower. Mo-Im Kim, in particular, viewed nurses' acquisition of leadership and management skills as central to this aim.[116] Her views were shared by others; three main articles in the *International Nursing Review* July/August 1990 issue focused on nurse management as a means to control health resource allocation. Written by British, American, and Australian authors, the articles contrasted sharply with Prem Mehra's "The Outlook for Nursing in India," which described a physician-dominated health care system unwilling to support nursing development on even the most basic level.[117] The disparity in nurse leadership development between nations was a potent reminder of the power of national politics over international ideals.

## Regulating Nursing

The disparately defined work and structure of nursing around the world prompted the ICN/FNIF-sponsored "Nursing Regulation: Moving Ahead" project in 1988. ICN leaders were concerned that lack of regulatory consensus in education, licensing, registration, and practice among NNAs detracted from nurses' power and participation in health care practice and policy. Six workshops on the Regulation of Nursing, funded by the W. K. Kellogg Foundation, Carnegie Corporation, British Overseas Development Administration, WHO, and Japanese and Korean Nursing Associations aimed to assist NNAs and their leaders to develop and implement national nursing regulatory systems reflective of international standards.

Held in different ICN regions between 1988 and 1991, the workshops were attended by 161 nurses from 99 NNAs and 62 government representatives. Nurses were encouraged to review, analyze, reassess, and participate in the revision of regulations and laws controlling nursing practice and care delivery in their countries.[118] In some countries, laws restricted nurses from their full scope of practice. In others, nurses practiced outside traditional boundaries of nurse practice without legal protection or regulation. In many instances, neither the nurse nor the public knew the extent

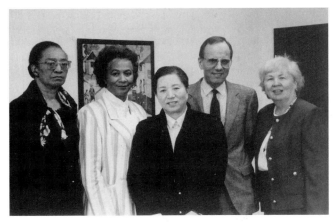

**FIGURE 5-18**
*At the ICN Offices in 1990. From left: Juanita Torres, Meryl
Hanson, President Mo-Im Kim, Trevor Clay, and Connie Hol-
leran. From ICN Collection.*

or limitation of nurse practice. Amelia Manglay-Maglacas, WHO chief
scientist for nursing, noted this problem in rural Africa and Asia: "Nurses
do almost anything and everything, including performing essential primary
surgery, suturing, and plastering fractured limbs . . . the disturbing fact is
that nurses do these tasks without prior training . . . many have learned
on the job and have become skillful."[119]

Nurses often performed acts traditionally assigned to physicians because of the lack of doctors. In some countries, midwives were particularly
vulnerable, carrying out breech deliveries, vacuum extraction and low
forceps delivery, extraction of retained placentas, blood transfusions, and
cesarean sections in the absence of medical support.[120] In other countries
where physicians dominated obstetrics practice, midwives were often rele-
gated to the margins of pregnancy and birth management. The difference
between midwifery practice among nations was broadly discussed at the
International Confederation of Midwives (ICM) meeting, Vancouver,
Canada in 1993.[121]

Holleran labeled the Regulation Project one of the "most significant
undertakings" of her 15-year administration. Without an official position
on international regulation of nursing practice, the ICN was vulnerable
to local governments, who could move into the vacuum and create nurse
practice acts more suited to political needs rather than professional standards.[122] Holleran urged the Council of National Representatives to study
nurse regulation and acquired funding from the W. K. Kellogg Foundation.
American Margretta Styles' earlier study and recommendation led the
1995 CNR to approve the project. Fadwa Affara was selected to direct
the 3-year Kellogg study with Dr. Styles as consultant.

# Worldwide Shortage

While regulation was a key ICN project in the early 1990s, immediate efforts to regulate nursing practice and education were overshadowed by critical shortages of nurses around the globe.[123] In 1990, for instance, the *Socio-Economic News* reported that Italian Health Minister Francesco de Lorenzo signed a decree permitting hospitals to recruit nursing staff from both inside and outside the European community. Claiming that Italy was "not getting value for its money under the present circumstances," de Lorenzo offered 37,000 jobs to foreign nurses as an emergency measure.[124]

The Federal Republic of Germany reported a crisis in nurse labor despite a national unemployment rate of 7%. Declining lengths of hospital stays (from 20.2 days in 1969 to 14.7 in 1989), increased nursing workloads through the use of technology and higher patient acuity, low wages, unattractive shift-work, and attrition through marriage and childbirth were identified as key contributors to the shortage. Officials soon looked to other countries to fill gaps in nurse supply.[125] Similar stories were reported in the United States, Canada, Great Britain, Australia, Israel, and other industrialized nations.

Nursing demand created by the AIDS epidemic in Zambia and other African nations was reported in field reports by ICN nurse consultants in the late 1980s.[126] Worldwide, sub-Saharan Africa was hardest hit by HIV/AIDS. In 1991, a reported 7 million adults and children were infected with the virus.[127] Amelia Manglay-Maglacas estimated that there were only 2.5 nurses per 10,000 individuals in Africa in 1989.[128]

With WHO funding, the ICN established a 2-year project to assist eight African members in their difficult battle against HIV/AIDS, complicated by congested wards and persistent shortages of staff and supplies. Efforts were made to educate nurses and the public about the virus, plan programs and services for the afflicted, and maintain up-to-date information on the status of the disease.[129]

Dr. Manglay-Maglacas of WHO blamed exacerbating global nurse shortage on the migration of nurses from developing to developed nations. The lure of high salaries and better working conditions, coupled with high-powered marketing, drew nurses away from their countries of origin and left critical nurse undersupply behind. Dr. Manglay-Maglacas was particularly sensitive to the massive emigration of nurses from her native Philippines. In 1989, 65% of the Island's 13,000 new nurse graduates from 132 nursing schools emigrated abroad, primarily to the United States and the Middle East.[130] The Philippines experienced a "brain drain" of nurse professionals that left its hospitals and community practices short-staffed.

On the other hand, the Irish Nurses Organisation discontinued participation in ICN's Nursing Abroad Program because of limited employment opportunities for foreign nurses.[131] Although Ireland denied a national nurse shortage, many Irish nurses emigrated in search of higher wages and

## THE END OF THE COLD WAR AND THE BEGINNING OF COLD WAR HISTORY

Kim's presidency coincided with the end of the Cold War, a term coined by *New York World* editor Herbert Bayard Swope to describe the post-World War II political and economic struggle between the capitalist, democratic Western powers and the communist Soviet Union. The Cold War period (1945–1991) was marked by massive military buildups (including nuclear arms) by both sides, intensive economic competition, and strained diplomatic relations. The first important disagreement between East and West concerned the reunification of Germany after East German authorities constructed a fortified wall across Berlin in August 1961. Communication between the two sides virtually ceased, and an "Iron Curtain" descended between them. To rally other Western powers behind its cause, the US sponsored a series of strategic actions, including the Marshall Plan and the North Atlantic Treaty Organization (NATO). Within the Communist bloc, the Soviet Union maintained tight political, economic, and military control over countries such as Hungary and Poland and supported Communist revolutions in China, parts of Southeast Asia, and Cuba. A period of eased tensions, known as Detente, occurred in the late 1960s and the 1970s, but the Soviet invasion of Afghanistan (1979) and US President Ronald Reagan's anti-Communist stance worsened relations between East and West. In the late 1980s and early 1990s Mikhail Gorbachev's policies diminished the power of hard-line Communists, and the USSR permitted the collapse of Communist regimes in Eastern Europe and the reunification of Germany in 1990. More cordial relations between the USSR and US led both nations' leaders to hail the end of the Cold War and the breakup of the Soviet Union in late 1991.

Based on John Lewis Gaddis, *We Now Know: Rethinking Cold War History*, Oxford: Clarendon Press, 1997.

better opportunity.[132] The Nordic countries boasted the highest nurse-to-population ratios in the world at between 85 and 87 per 10,000.[133] Like the Irish Nurses Organisation, the Norwegian Nurses Association announced its plan to terminate its Nursing Abroad program due to job unavailability for foreign exchangees.

Although ICN recognized individuals' right to relocate, it worried that migration thwarted local and international efforts to improve short-term nurse recruitment and retention and long-term personnel planning. The Council of National Representatives committed ICN to assisting member associations to study nursing personnel needs and resources, share information pertaining to nursing's worldwide employment status, and continue discussion of the international impact of nurse shortage. In its report to the 42nd World Health Assembly (WHA), Geneva, Switzerland, 1989, ICN urged WHO's member states to review their national nursing/midwifery needs and resources; develop strategies to recruit, retain, educate, and reorient nurses and midwives; elevate nurses to senior health leadership and management positions; support research pertaining to nursing; and adopt health policies to facilitate nurse/midwife participation in primary care.[134]

Meanwhile, the American Nurses Association (ANA) successfully lobbied against the American Medical Association's (AMA) plan to solve critical nurse undersupply through the creation of the "registered care technician" (RCT). The RCT, a newly created health care worker, would be trained through AMA-sponsored programs to assist professional nurses. Many nurses feared that the new worker, under medicine's educational control but nursing's clinical supervision, would redefine nursing practice and add additional responsibilities to already overworked nursing staff.

The ANA also attempted to preserve nurse practice standards threatened by new payment systems based on prospective payment and diagnosis-related groups (DRGs). DRGs categorized hospitalized patients by principal diagnosis, age, sex, complicating conditions, and the presence or absence of surgical intervention to predetermine the amount of money necessary for their care. Based exclusively on a medical model, DRGs did not reflect the actual or potential nursing resources or time devoted to patient care in various categories. The ANA struggled to maintain control of nursing in an environment chiefly concerned with the economics of medical health care delivery.[135]

## Naming Nursing Care

In 1989, based on these developments at home, the ANA proposed a council resolution that urged their fellow NNAs to monitor local changes in health care service payments and their impact on nursing. From this information, it was proposed, NNAs could develop country-specific classification systems for nursing care that would then be translated internationally.[136]

ANA argued that, unless nursing could name its distinct contribution to health care, the profession's work would continue to go unrecognized in worldwide health care planning and financing. Collecting and documenting data on nursing practice across clinical settings, client populations, geographic borders, and time would assist in planning types and amounts of nursing and health service, determining skill mixes for different care settings and client groups, and evaluating clinical practice efficacy and cost.

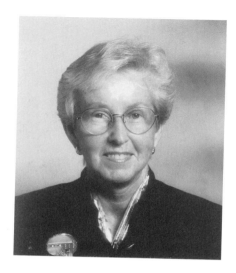

**FIGURE 5-19**

*Margretta Styles, ICN President 1993 to 1997. From ICN Collection.*

In 1990, as a follow-up to the ANA-proposed CNR resolution, the ICN Board of Directors invited June Clark (UK) and Norma Lang (US) to develop a feasibility study for an International Classification for Nursing Practice (ICNP) along with Margretta[16] Madden Styles, chair of the Professional Services Committee, Fadwa Affara,[17] and Denmark's Randi Mortenson and Gunnar Nielsen.[18] Over the next 7 years, in consultation with nurses and classification experts, the team collected, grouped, and ranked nursing phenomena, interventions, and outcomes and developed architecture to define their interrelationships.[137] As did Isabel Hampton Robb in 1909, the team aimed to create a Nursing Esperanto that would create a universal nursing language.

In 1993, American Margretta Madden Styles was voted the ICN's 22nd president at the Council of National Representatives Meeting in Madrid, Spain. With an organization 110 members strong comprising 1.4 million nurses, Styles assumed leadership still chiefly concerned with matters related to professional services' issues, economic stability, international relations, and global nurse representation.

Between 1989 and 1993, the ICN lost 2 longstanding members, India and Australia, as the result of dues-related issues, but gained 14. Resolutions were passed to promote nursing research, nurse entrepreneurship, and nurses' occupational safety; protect patients from chemicals and pesticides, toxic waste, and inhumane care; and encourage the education of female children.[138] Recommendations issued to NNAs supported the development of culturally appropriate and sensitive mental health/psychiatric nursing models for education and practice.

## Blueprint for the Future

Adopting "Toward the 21st Century: A Strategic Plan, 1994–1999" at the 1993 CNR meeting created a new blueprint for future ICN activities. Sounding some familiar and some new themes, the plan committed ICN to formulating health and social policy, worldwide professional standardization and socioeconomic equity for nurses, collaboration with other international organizations around areas of mutual concern, increased membership, dissemination of nursing knowledge, and the development of frameworks for gathering and measuring nurses' work.[139]

The Strategic Plan's significance lies in its explicit "priority work," described by Styles as a means "to make more systematic and clear and open the processes for arriving at critical decisions about what *should* and what *can* be accomplished with limited resources."[140] The ICN developed a long-term financial plan for management of its activities. Part of the plan involved a proposed per capita dues increase of 1% in 1998 and 1% in 1999.

An ICN Board Task Force was established to examine structural and organizational issues that might interfere with the proposed Strategic Plan. Cochaired by Gay Williams (New Zealand) and Tassana Boontong (Thailand), the task force sent out questionnaires to all NNAs in May 1994 to determine their positions on select criteria: ICN membership, NNA recruitment and retention, dues policy, voting procedures and rights, and ICN Board representation. Analyzing the responses of the 60 returned questionnaires, the task force made several key recommendations to the Council of National Representatives in these areas.

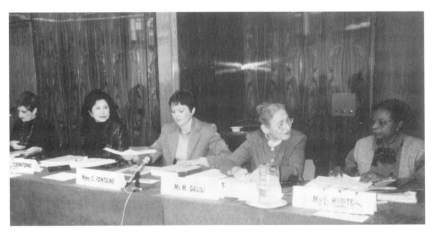

**FIGURE 5-20**
*ICN Board (1994). From left: Alice Baumgart, Tassana Boontong, Cecile Fontaine, Moriah Galili, and Eleane Hunte. From ICN Collection.*

| ICN Board Task Force Proposal for Weighted Voting for NNAs | | |
|---|---|---|
| Numbers of Members | Number of Votes | NNAs in Category |
| 0–5,000 | 1 | 88 |
| 5–10,000 | 2 | 6 |
| 10–50,000 | 3 | 10 |
| Over 50,000 | 4 | 6 |

The issue of NNA voting rights was raised as a particular concern. Questions resurfaced about continuation of the one vote–one NNA policy. The task force proposed a system of weighted voting that allocated numbers of votes in accordance with numbers of members.

Of the NNA responses to the proposed system of weighted voting, 10 found the system "highly desirable," 17 "acceptable," 6 "worthy of consideration," 20 "not acceptable," 7 needed more information, and 1 did not respond. Concerns expressed by those opposed to the measure included that smaller associations would be underrepresented at CNR, that the ICN membership would be focused on individuals rather than NNAs, and that weighting larger associations would minimize equitable power distribution. The 50 associations that did not respond likely fell into the smallest member category. Ultimately, the system of one voting representative per NNA at CNR was retained. The issue of weighted voting was deferred to a later time, but the open discussion of the matter was well received by the CNR.

The ICN endorsed several position statements at the 1995 CNR meeting in Harare, Zimbabwe. Revisiting its 1981 Resolution on Female Excision, Circumcision and Mutilation (FGM), the organization resolved to take a more active position in eliminating FGM through cooperation with local, national, and international groups opposed to the practice.[141] Position statements pertaining to mental health/psychiatric nursing and the costs and value of nursing were also endorsed.[142] Resolutions were proposed that addressed titling, nursing's participation in health policy, guidelines for accreditation of systems for schools of nursing, competition in health services, cultural safety, and the role of nursing students in NNAs.

Holleran's final report to the CNR reflected a healthy ICN headed toward the 21st century. One hundred and ten members strong, the ICN set its sights on continuing efforts to influence health and social policy, maintain quality professional and socioeconomic standards, and empower NNAs to act on the behalf of their nations' nurses. Holleran encouraged ICN members to continue to document their work, become active participants in local and international health matters, and maintain communication between associations and international bodies. Although speaking about the last 5 years of her tenure, she could just as well have reflected on the ICN's 96-year history in her comment, "I hope you can agree that we have come a long way quickly for such a diverse group."[143]

## ENDNOTES

1. "ICN Profile of an International Nursing Leader," *The Philippine Journal of Nursing,* 42 (January–March 1973): 34–35. Kruse served as chair of the EPN from 1948 to 1961 and as a member of SEW from 1961 to 1965.

2. Circular letter to the ICN Board of Directors from Margrethe Kruse, 12 August 1969, pp. 1–6, ICNA. The inability to maintain staff was particularly due to the "exceedingly low" salaries for the amount of work, time, and effort expected from and expended by the small staff. Helen Nussbaum's ill health forced her early retirement on December 31, 1967. Sheila Quinn succeeded Nussbaum as executive secretary on January 1, 1968.

3. "News from ICN," *International Nursing Review,* 13 (July/August, 1966): 4.

4. Kruse wrote to the board that Quinn's resignation was "not a surprise" because Quinn had informed her at Kruse's first visit to Geneva in July 1969 that "she intended to apply for a position in England when an opportunity offered." See circular letter to ICN Board of Directors from Margrethe Kruse, 24 November 1969, ICNA.

5. Circular letter to the ICN Board of Directors from Margrethe Kruse, May 1970, p. 2, ICNA.

6. Herwitz was paid SF 6,500 per month, a figure almost double that paid Quinn. Kruse justified this sum on "account of the temporary nature of the appointment and the extra expenses incurred by having to maintain a home in two places." Circular letter to the ICN Board of Directors from Margrethe Kruse, 5 March 1970, ICNA.

7. "ICN Executive Director Appointed," News Release, No. 13, 9 October 1970, ICNA.

8. Grace Murabito Thomas, "Nursing in Lebanon," *International Nursing Review,* 22 (September/October 1975): 138–143.

9. "Report of the ICN Executive Director to the Council of National Representatives," May 1973, Mexico City, Mexico, p. 2, ICNA.

10. Adele Herwitz, CHART (The Official Publication of the Illinois Nurses' Association, USA), 69 (February 1972): 40.

11. Rene Maheu, director-general UNESCO, "Resolution 8 Adopted by the General Conference at Its Sixteenth Session" (October–November 1970), form letter sent to ICN, 14 January 1971, "South African Material . . . ," ICNA.

12. For a comprehensive history of South African nursing, see Shula Marks, *Divided Sisterhood: Race, Class and Gender in the South African Nursing Profession* (New York: St. Martin's Press, 1994).

13. Gunvor Stjernlof, executive secretary Swedish Nurses Association to ICN Board of Directors, 28 November 1972, "South African Material . . . ," ICNA.

14. John E. Fobes to Adele Herwitz, 2 August 1972, p. 1–3, in "South African Material Used for ICN History, 1970–1972," ICNA. The ICN was one of several organizations suspended by UNESCO because of UNESCO's policy against apartheid and racial discrimination.

15. Adele Herwitz to P. H. Harrison, 17 April 1972, "South African . . . ," ICNA.

16. D. H. Radloff, South African Nurses Association, to Adele Herwitz, 25 May 1972, Enclosure with circular letter from headquarters, July 1972, ICNA.

17. Circular letter to ICN Board of Directors from Adele Herwitz, July 1972, "South African . . . ," ICNA.

18. Minutes of the Meeting of the Board of Directors, 9–11 May 1973, Mexico City, Mexico, p. 13, ICNA.

19. Minutes of the Meeting of the Board of Directors, 9–11 May 1973, Mexico City, Mexico, "Memorandum to the Board of Directors of the International Council of Nurses from the Board of the South African Nursing Association," Annex 1, pp. 23–26, ICNA. Numbers of nonwhite nurses rose from 546 in 1948 to over 17,000 in 1972.

20. Barbara Beal "Bantu Nursing," *American Journal of Nursing,* 70 (March 1970): 547–550. Beal was the health coordinator of Up With People, Inc., an organization providing health care to individuals traveling abroad in educational programs. It is unclear why she made the South African trip.

21. Ibid., 14; "South African Nurses Called on to End Discrimination or Face Expulsion from ICN," *International Nursing Review,* 20 (July/August 1973): 101–102.

22. The board did not support SANA's expulsion because there was no specific breech in the standards of ICN membership.

23. "Withdrawal of the South African Nursing Association from the International Council of Nurses: Summary of a Talk Given by Miss P. H. Harrison, Vice-President of the South African Nursing Association, 8 August 1973," *South African Nursing Journal,* 40 (September 1973): 7–8. Harrison attributed the undue burden of dues payment to SANA's withdrawal.

24. Michael Bangs, "Ungraceful Withdrawal," *Nursing Times,* 69 (November 15, 1973): 1505.

25. A. F. S. Towert, Letter to the Editor, *South African Nursing Journal,* 40 (December 1973): 13.

26. Ibid.

27. Fifteen years later, on 16 August 1988, American Public Health Association Executive Director William H. McBeath wrote to ICN Executive Director Constance Holleran to recommend ICN sever ties with SANA because of South Africa's apartheid policy, apparently unaware that they had done so already. Letter to Constance Holleran from William H. McBeath, ICNA.

28. "Nurses Say 'No' to Smoking," *International Nursing Review,* 20, 5 (September–October 1973): 135.

29. Dorothy S. Starr, "ICN Meets in Mexico," *The Canadian Nurse,* 69 (August 1973): 22 and "ICN Supports Non-Smoking Action," *The Philippines Journal of Nursing,* 42, 3 (July–September 1973): 179.

30. The ICN and ILO had a longstanding relationship around issues pertaining to nurses' employment conditions. See Adele Herwitz, "An International Look at Employment Problems," *American Journal of Nursing,* 59, 3 (March 1959): 355–357.

31. "Circular Letter from Headquarters: To the ICN Board of Directors from Adele Herwitz," Number 4 (June 1974), ICNA.

32. ICN Report of the Executive Director to the CNR, May 1977, Tokyo, Japan, "ICN Programme 1975–1977," p. 9, ICNA.

33. Minutes of the Council of National Representatives Meeting, "ICN Report of the President to the Council of National Representatives," May 1977, Tokyo, Japan, Annex J, Agenda Item 9, p. 3, ICNA.

34. Dorothy Cornelius, "Report of the ICN President, 1973–1975," *International Nursing Review* (September/October 1975): 168.

35. Minutes of the Board of Directors, ICN "Accounts," 31 December 1975, Annex Q, Agenda Item 16.1, ICNA.

36. Margrethe Kruse, "Confrontation with a Quadrennium," *International Nursing Review*, 21, 3 (March/April 1974): 82.
37. Dorothy Cornelius, "Report of the ICN President, 1973–1975," *International Nursing Review*, 22 (September/October 1975): 174.
38. Starr, "ICN Meets in Mexico," 18.
39. Margrethe Kruse, "ICN at the Crossroads," *International Nursing Review*, 20 (March/April 1973): 43 (42–46).
40. Ibid.
41. "Definition of Nurse," *International Nursing Review*, 21 (March/April 1974): 103.
42. Ibid.
43. Minutes of the Meeting of the Council of National Representatives, 1969, "Report on the Position of Auxiliary Nursing Personnel in Relation to Membership in National Nurses Associations," Agenda Item 15a, Annex 10, pp. 1–6, ICNA.
44. ICN National Reports of Member Associations, 1973, "Japan," ICNA. Reports of national nurses associations in ICN membership were first published in 1957. Every 4 years, at the time of ICN's quadrennial congresses, a new edition of the National Reports of Member Associations was prepared.
45. Akiko Takahashi, "The Changing Status of Nursing as a Profession in Japan," *The Nursing Journal of Singapore*, 20 (August 1980): 68–71. Takahashi, director of nursing services at Osaka Prefectural, Senri Critical Care Medical Center, presented an overview of Japanese nursing history at the Singapore-Japan Nursing Symposium 28–30 July 1980.
46. For an excellent review of Japanese nursing history, see Kay K. Hisama, "Florence Nightingale's Influence on the Development and Professionalization of Modern Nursing in Japan," *Nursing Outlook*, 44, 6 (1996): 284–288.
47. See Minutes of the Council of National Representatives, 1969, "Report on the Position of Auxiliary Nursing Personnel in Relation to Membership in National Associations," Annex 8, Agenda Item 15a, pp. 1–6, ICNA.
48. Starr, "ICN Meets in Mexico," 22.
49. Minutes of the Meeting of the Council of National Representatives, 12–15, 17 May 1973, Mexico City, Mexico, "To Consider and Take Action on a Proposal for an Increase in ICN Dues," Agenda Item 20, Annex 5, pp. 38–39, ICNA.
50. Canada reported 104,124 members, Japan 143,766, and the United States 173,990 in 1975. The next largest organization, the United Kingdom, reported 45,566 members. Dorothy Cornelius, "Report of the ICN President, 1973–1975," *International Nursing Review*, 22 (September/October 1975): 175.
51. For discussions of nursing in Senegal, Paraguay, and Mozambique, see Ibrahima Dieng, "Evolution of the Nursing Profession in Senegal, " *International Nursing Review*, 21, 6 (November/December 1974): 172–173; Marcelina Palacios de Gomez, "Nursing in Paraguay," *International Nursing Review*, 25, 2 (March/April 1978): 48–50; and Christine Webb, "A New Nursing Education Programme for Independent Mozambique," *International Nursing Review*, 26, 2 (March/April 1979): 41–48.
52. Minutes of the Council of National Representatives Meeting, May 1977, "Report of the President to the CNR," Annex J, Agenda Item 9, p. 9, ICNA.
53. Circular letter to the ICN Board of Directors from Adele Herwitz, November 1975, "Field Work," p. 2, ICNA. Herwitz discusses field visits to Malta and Indonesia by other ICN staff during this period that did not "come to fruition."
54. Starr, "ICN Meets in Mexico," 18.

55. Dorothy Cornelius, "Report of the ICN President, 1973–1975," *International Nursing Review*, 22 (September/October 1975): 168.

56. *The RCN and the ICN*, p. 1–13, ICNA.

57. Ibid., 2.

58. Adele Herwitz to ICN Board of Directors, circular letter from headquarters, May 1975, No. 1, p. 1, ICNA.

59. Cornelius, "Report of the ICN President, 1973–1975," 172.

60. See correspondence to Dorothy Cornelius from W. E. Prentice (Royal College of Nursing President), 16 July 1975, *Specific Issues of Particular Significance to the RCN*, p. 1–3, "RCN Materials Used for 1964–1965 History," ICNA.

61. "Rough" notes of "Meeting Held at RCN Headquarters, London, UK, With Officials of RCN at the Request of President of ICN, February 7, 1975," Verna Splane to Dorothy Cornelius, 15 February 1975, ICNA.

62. Catherine M. Hall (RCN general secretary) to Adele Herwitz, 1 December 1975, "Materials for RCN . . . ," ICNA. 1,747 voted to rescind, 569 to support the withdrawal resolution.

63. A. Mejia, H. Pizurki, and E. Royston. *Physician and Nurse Migration: Analysis and Policy Implications* (Geneva: World Health Organization, 1979).

64. For an in-depth discussion of the migration patterns of nurses from the Philippines to US hospitals in particular, see Barbara L. Brush. Sending for Nurses: Foreign Nurse Immigration to American Hospitals, 1945–1980. (PhD dissertation, University of Pennsylvania, 1994).

65. Dame Sheila Quinn, *ICN Past and Present* (London: Scutari Press, 1989). Quinn describes her personal experience with the earlier transaction on pp. 127–129.

66. Adele Herwitz to ICN Board of Directors, circular letter from headquarters, November 1975, "Legacy from Christiane Reimann," p. 3, ICNA.

67. Adele Herwitz to ICN Board of Directors, circular letter from headquarters, June 1976, "The Christiane Reimann Story—Next Chapter," p. 1–2, ICNA.

68. Dorothy Cornelius, "ICN Watchword," *International Nursing Review*, 24, 5 (September/October 1977): 152.

69. Ibid.

70. *Socio-Economic News*, written by the executive director, began in February 1980 and appeared every 2 months.

71. See Foreword, Sheila Quinn (Ed.), *What About Me? Caring for the Carers* (Geneva: International Council of Nurses, 1981).

72. Cited by Doris Krebs, "Report of the Symposium on 'Nursing in Primary Care: Strategies for Action,'" Los Angeles, California, 2 July 1981, ICNA.

73. "ICN States Support of Primary Health Care," *International Nursing Review*, 26, 1 (January/February 1979): 3–4.

74. Minutes of the Council of National Representatives, A. Mangay-Maglacas, "ICN Symposium, Los Angeles, 2 July 1981: Strategies for Health for All," Annex I, ICNA.

75. Minutes of the Council of National Representatives, "Resolution Proposed by the Members Association of Australia: Female Excision, Circumcision and Mutilation," Annex N, 9 September 1980, ICNA. A cost analysis of circumcision was done by WHO advisor Fran Hosken. Hosken highlighted such "costs" as the loss of life, necessary hospitalization secondary to infection, childbirth hazards, work time lost to illness, and the operation costs associated with the procedure.

76. Fran P. Hosken, *The Hosken Report*, 3rd rev. ed. (Lexington, MA: Women's International Network News, 1982). Hosken noted 3 years later that, despite

worldwide attention to the problem, little had changed. However, in 1990, the Organization of African Unity adopted The African Charter on the Rights and Welfare of the Child that made it mandatory for governments to take active measures to eliminate "harmful traditional social and cultural practices affecting children." See Robbi Robson, "The Issue of Unspoken Abuse," *Nursing Standard*, 4, 8 (May 1994): 16–17.

77. ICN Minutes of the Post-Council of National Representatives Meeting of the Board of Directors, 4–5 June 1977, Tokyo, Japan, Agenda Item 19, ICNA and Krebs, "Report of the Symposium."

78. Craig Little, "Inside ICN Headquarters With Constance Holleran," *Nursing and Health Care*, 11, 8 (October 1990): 406–410. Holleran facilitated the successful organization of nurses across the United States to become a strong force in achieving more adequate funding for health and social programs, chairing the Coalition for Health Funding with its representative 50 health-related groups.

79. Interview, Constance Holleran by Joan E. Lynaugh and Barbara L. Brush, Center for the Study of the History of Nursing, University of Pennsylvania, School of Nursing, Philadelphia, Pennsylvania, 20 June 1994, Transcript, p. 6.

80. Minutes of the ICN Board of Directors, 27 June 1981, Los Angeles, California, USA, "Executive Director's Report, 15 March–June 1981," p. 6, Annex 2, Agenda Item 5, ICNA.

81. Helen K. Mussallem, "Continuing Education: An Essential to Nursing Strategy and Networks in Primary Health Care," A Commonwealth Foundation Lectureship in West Africa and Mediterranean (London: The Commonwealth Foundation, 1981), 22.

82. Anstey died suddenly 2 years after leaving office. "Olive Anstey Dies," *International Nursing Review*, 30, 5 (September/October 1983): 131.

83. *Socio-Economic News*, no. 1, February 1980, ICNA.

84. See Sheila Quinn (Ed.), *What About Me?* and *Cooperation and Conflict* in the Caring for the Carers series (Geneva: International Council of Nurses, 1981 and 1983).

85. Constance Holleran, Executive Director's Report, 1985, ICNA.

86. Interview, Constance Holleran, transcript, p. 54.

87. Memorandum to ICN Nurse Advisors from Juanita C. Torres, Business Manager, 12 September 1985, ICNA.

88. Jenny Gibbs, "Let Justice Be Done," *The Australian Nurses Journal*, 15, 3 (August 1985): 5.

89. Nelly Garzon, Acceptance Speech, ICN Congress, Tel Aviv, Israel, 1985, ICNA.

90. "Nurses Can Spark Social Change, Say ICN Speakers," *The American Nurse*, 17, 7 (July/August 1985): 19.

91. Letter to Constance Holleran from J. L. Gibbs, RANF president, 21 June 1985, ICNA.

92. Letter from Constance Holleran to J. L. Gibbs, 23 January 1986, ICNA.

93. Constance Holleran, "Greetings to the World Conference of Health Workers on Social Well-Being, Health and Peace," 5 June 1987, Moscow, USSR, ICNA.

94. Interview, Constance Holleran, transcript, p. 29.

95. Richard Wells, Peggy Nutall, and WHO, "AIDS," *International Nursing Review*, 32, 3 (May/June 1985): 76–79, 83. Quotation is on p. 79.

96. Letter to Constance Holleran, 5 April 1985, ICNA.

97. Letter from Constance Holleran to Mrs. Nancy Gibson, 24 November 1986, ICNA.

98. Andrew Whitley, "Striking Nurses Challenge Israeli Policy on Wages," *Financial Times*, 8 July 1986, 7.

99. Constance Holleran, "Report of the Field Visit to the Trained Nurses' Association of India," 10–14 February 1986, ICNA.

100. Translated letter to Nelly Garzon from Marta Aravena Vidal, 15 April 1986, ICNA. The nurses, Mrs. Corral and Mrs. Reush, were released on bail 1 month before the letter was written.

101. No doubt too, Holleran must have been concerned with keeping associations in membership happy; in 1987, 2.2 million SF of the ICN's 1987 2.5 million SF income was generated by membership dues. See "ICN Financial Budget 1986–1987" as addendum to the board of directors, "1986/1987 Proposed Programme Budget," Agenda Item 8.3.2, ICN Minutes of the Board of Directors, 1986, ICNA.

102. Constance Holleran, "Report of a Field Visit to Taiwan (The Nurses Association of the Republic of China)," 11–13 May 1986, ICNA.

103. Constance Holleran, "Field Visit Report: Chinese Nursing Association," 24–28 May 1988, ICNA.

104. Letter to Constance Holleran from Tung-Ling Ma, 19 May 1990, ICNA.

105. Mireille Kingma, "Report of Field Visit to Cote d'Ivoire," 24–28 January 1988, ICNA.

106. Helga Morrow, "Report of Field Visit to the Nurses Association of Malta," 21–27 April 1987, ICNA.

107. Taka Oguisso estimated that only 5% or 150 nurses in Guatemala were members of the professional association. See Taka Oguisso, "Report of Field Visit to Asociacion Guatemalteca de Enfermeras Profesionales," 24–31 January 1988 and "Report of Field Visit to Asociacion Nacional de Enfermeras Salvadorenas, 31 January–5 February 1988, ICNA. The Salvadorean National Nurses Association had been an ICN member since 1969.

108. Helga Morrow, "Report of Field Visit to the Lesotho Nurses' Association," 22–27 February 1988, ICNA. The Kingdom of Lesotho, formerly Basutoland, gained its independence from Great Britain on October 4, 1966.

109. Mireille Kingma, "Report of Field Visit to Association Nationale des Infirmiers et Infirmieres Diplomes d'Etat du Senegal," 12–17 January 1988, p. 2, ICNA.

110. Memorandum from Juanita C. Torres, business manager to the ICN Board of Directors re: 1st Quarter Financial Report for 1988, April 1988, ICNA.

111. Memorandum to ICN Board of Directors from Juanita C. Torres, business manager, 4th Quarter Financial Report 1988, February 1989, ICNA.

112. ICN Minutes, "ICN Financial Budget 1986–1987," p. 2, ICNA.

113. ICN Board of Directors Minutes 1986/1987, "Proposed Budget," Agenda Item 8.3.2, BD 1986, p. 5, ICNA. Of the remaining income, SF 2.2 million came from dues payments, 153,750 from interests and dividends, 70,000 from publication sales, 1,000 from royalties, and 10,000 from miscellaneous sources.

114. Letter to NNAs from Mo-Im Kim, December 1989, ICNA.

115. Dame Nita Barrow, "Nursing—A New Tomorrow," *International Nursing Review*, 36, 5 (May 1989): 143.

116. Mo-Im Kim, "Making ICN a Catalyst of Change," *International Nursing Review*, 36, 6 (June 1989): 171–173.

117. Christine Hancock, "Making the Case for Nurses as Managers of Health Services": 105–108; Joyce C. Kadandara, "Making the Case for Nurses as Managers of Nursing Resources": 109–112; Dorothy J. del Bueno, "Preparation of Nurse Managers": 117–120; and Prem Mehra, "The Outlook for Nursing in India": 121–122 are all in *International Nursing Review*, 36, 4 (July/August 1990).

118. Minutes of Council of National Representatives, Agenda Item 10, p. 3, Items 18–20, ICNA.

119. Amelia Mangay-Maglacas, "Close Encounters in International Nursing: Impact on Health Policy and Research," *Journal of Professional Nursing*, 5, 6 (November–December 1989): 311.

120. ICM/WHO/UNICEF. *Statement of the ICM/WHO/UNICEF Pre-Congress Workshop on Midwifery Education—Action for Safe Motherhood*. Kobe, Japan, 1990.

121. Papers given at the ICM Congress, Vancouver, 1993 on this subject included H. M. McCoker, "Barriers to Diversity in Caring for the Childbearing Family," J. M. Carlson and J. M. O'Heir, "Midwives of the Future: Preventing the Medicalization of Childbirth in the Developing World," Brian Burtch, "Trial of Labour: Midwifery Practice and Legal Regulation," and C. Benoit, "Conceptualizing Care in the Personnel Service Professions: The Case of Female Health Practitioners."

122. Interview, Constance Holleran, transcript, p. 51.

123. Minutes of the Council of National Representatives, "Executive Director's Report," 1991, Agenda Item 8.2, pp. 1–7, ICNA.

124. *Socio-economic News*, No. 91, October 1990, pp. 2–3.

125. This information, presented in the March 1990 issue of *Socio-Economic News*, No. 85, p. 2, was synthesized from German sources: *Die Welt* (Bonn) 11 and 14 July 1989; *Badische Neueste Nachrichten*, 8 and 11 August 1989; and *Munchner Merkur* (Munich) 26 and 28 July 1989.

126. Helga Morrow, "Report of Field Visit to the National Nurses Association of Kenya (NNAK)," 2–9 and 18–19 August 1989, ICNA; Morrow, "Report of Field Visit With the Zambia Nurses' Association," 26 July–2 August 1989, ICNA.

127. WHO Press Release, 28 November 1991. Reprinted in Joan MacNeil, "Sharing the Challenge: Mobilizing Nurses Against HIV/AIDS in Africa," *International Nursing Review*, 39 (May/June 1992): 77–82.

128. Amelia Manglay-Maglacas, "Close Encounters in International Nursing": 310.

129. "Mobilizing Nurses for AIDS Prevention and Care in Eight African Countries" was earmarked for Cote d'Ivoire, Ghana, Malawi, Tanzania, Togo, Uganda, Zaire, and Zambia.

130. Senator Neptali A. Gonzales, "Let Us Nurse Our Society Back to Health," *Philippine Journal of Nursing*, 59 (July–September, 1989): 11–14. Gonzales also questioned the continued rapid production of nurses and the emphasis of their training. Of the 35% nurses remaining in the Philippines, over half worked in urban hospitals even though the country's major health problems were among the rural poor.

131. Letter to Constance Holleran from Hilary Marchant, deputy general secretary, The Irish Nurses Organisation, 15 August 1989, ICNA.

132. This was reported by Katherine McInerney in "Report of Field Visit to the Irish Nurses Organisation and National Council of Nurses of Ireland," 22–27 October 1989, ICNA.

133. Amelia Manglay-Maglacas, "Close Encounters in International Nursing": 310.

134. World Health Association Resolution, "Strengthening Nursing and Midwifery in Support of Strategies for Health for All," reprinted in *International Nursing Review*, 36 (May 1989): 104.

135. For a more complete discussion of changes in the American health care system, see Joan E. Lynaugh and Barbara L. Brush, *American Nursing: From Hospitals to Health Systems* (Cambridge, MA and Oxford, UK: Blackwell Publishers, 1996).

136. Minutes of the Council of National Representatives, CNR Resolution, "Payment Systems Based on Prospective Payment and Diagnosis-Related Groups," 1989, Annex Agenda Item 12.7, ICNA.
137. For a more complete understanding of the ICNP, see "Introducing ICN's International Classification for Nursing Practice (ICNP): A Unifying Framework": 169–170; June Clark, "How Nurses Can Participate in the Development of an ICNP": 171–174; Gunnar H. Nielson and Randi A. Mortensen, "The Architecture for an International Classification for Nursing Practice (ICNP)": 175–182; Amy Coenen and Madeline Wake, "Developing a Database for an International Classification for Nursing Practice (ICNP)": 183–187; and "ICNP in Europe: Telenurse": 188–189 in *International Nursing Review*, 43, 6 (June 1996).
138. Minutes of the Meeting of the Council of National Representatives, 21–23 June 1993, Madrid, Spain, Annex D-R, ICNA.
139. See Minutes of the Council of National Representatives, Documents, Harare, Zimbabwe, September 1995, pp. 27–40, ICNA for a detailed discussion of ICN strategy areas, contributory activities, and outcomes between 1993 and 1995.
140. International Council of Nurses, Council of National Representatives, Harare, Zimbabwe, September 1995, "Report of the President," Agenda Item 7.1, p. 17, ICNA.
141. Groups identified in the Position Statement included The Inter-African Committee on Traditional Practices Affecting the Health of Women and Children (IAC); the Foundation for Women's Health, Research and Development (FORWARD); and the International Planned Parenthood Foundation.
142. Minutes of the Council of National Representatives, Harare, Zimbabwe, September 1995, Annex 2, 3, and 4, pp. 59–65, ICNA.
143. Minutes of the Meeting of the Council of National Representatives, September 1995, "Executive Director's Report," Agenda Item 7.2, p. 23, ICNA.

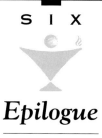

# *Epilogue*

BARBARA L. BRUSH and JOAN E. LYNAUGH
*for the ICN History Collective*

*A*s we reflect on this 100-year history of innovation, growth, change, conflict, and resolution, we revisit the five central themes guiding our interpretation: the ICN's shifting identity; its ability to survive as an organization; its responses to class, race, and gender differences; the changing definition of nurses' work and worth; and the relationships between nurses across cultures and nations. These perspectives help us understand an organization of nurses whose century-old struggles, compromises, and victories helped shape the occupation of nursing and the work of nurses around the globe.

As we have seen, the ICN's change from an "imagined community" of a few homogeneous nurse reformers to a conglomerate of nurses with different cultural, racial, ethnic, religious, and social backgrounds challenged early leaders' assumptions about the universality of nurses' work and female values. Is nursing universal? The ICN has always said "yes," but the meaning of universality has changed over time. Nurses demanded that the ICN take on new perspectives and initiate bolder, perhaps unpopular stances in the face of pressing humanitarian issues. The ICN has fought against racial discrimination, female genital mutilation, child abuse, nuclear proliferation, human rights abuses, and many other worldwide problems. Taking positions on issues outside of nursing's immediate occupational realm demonstrates the ICN's evolution from a professional rule-making association to an international policy-making body.

Part of this shift can be attributed to the growing strength of self-determination and free choice among nurses. The movement away from the idea of a collective authority to individual self-determination also constituted a change in the meaning of the word unity as originally used by Fenwick.[1] Instead, as ICN leaders like Margrethe Kruse saw it, the concept of unity meant like-minded people pursuing similar ends in their own ways—powerfully linked together by shared interests. One requirement for implementing self-determination was better general education for all; it seems that a more equitable imagined community coincided with better general education for more women in the world.

Recent ICN initiatives toward universality in nursing, such as the work on professional regulation and the International Classification of Nursing Practice, suggest growing consensus around idea sharing in place of the founders' exhortations to a single line of professional ideology and behavior.[2] None of this, however, intends to suggest that these changes always worked in a single direction, nor, because they reflect the style of certain leaders, are they immutable. Still, we found significant alteration in basic ICN thinking about how humans relate to one another and how humanity is best organized to care for the sick. New resolutions passed at the 1997 CNR meeting reflect this continuing trend: collaboration between national nurse associations and national organizations of physicians, prevention programs against sexual violence, ensuring workplace safety, the ethical implications of cloning in terms of human health, and unfettered reappraisal of nursing history and the dissemination of historical research on nursing.[3]

The organization's transformation from a sisterhood of like-minded women to a corporation of 120 national associations and a million and a half members also helps account for its survival in the international arena. Its expanding size and funded projects translated into greater financial security and, with that, greater power and self-confidence. Growth continues today. In 1997, the Democratic Nursing Organization of South Africa and Australia's College of Nursing began to represent their nations at the ICN along with new representative groups from Brazil, Romania, and Slovakia.[4] Associations from The Republic of Georgia, Vietnam, Indonesia, Macedonia, Saudi Arabia, Iran, Rwanda, and Gabon will likely be admitted at the 1999 Council of National Representatives (CNR) meeting in London. Celebrating and symbolizing its self-concept as a "new corporate identity," the ICN launched its new logo at the June 1997 Vancouver Congress. The new blue and yellow design uses a core figure and symbols of balance, light, and universality to depict the nurse working with people. The logo is also intended to mark a flexible and receptive modern organization prepared to tackle a new millennium.

Despite the organization's attention to wider world issues, the desire on the part of nurses for recognition of their work remains central, and perhaps little changed, in ICN's *raison d'être*. Today's efforts to name and quantify the work of nurses in relationship to care and costs, establish regulatory standards, prepare nurse leaders, address worklife issues, and reform health care have high priority.[5] These imperatives often coincide with the "special" needs of women around the globe: socioeconomic welfare and security, personal health and safety, and human rights. Indeed, the long life of the ICN demonstrates the potency and appeal of women collecting around common interests.

As such, the ICN reflects the history of women. Men in nursing moved onto the ICN stage as the organization became more universal. The significance of men as ICN members was sharply recognized in the 1961 argument between the ICN and the International Labour Organization (ILO), which wanted to label the ICN as a "women's organization." In recent decades, men have become CNR representatives and taken on leadership roles in national

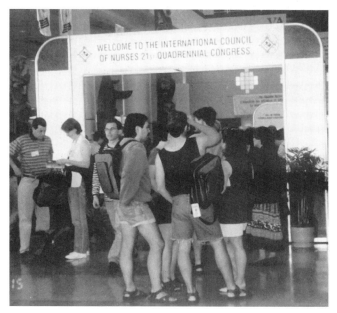

**FIGURE 6-1**
*Registering at the 1997 ICN Congress in Vancouver, British Columbia, Canada. From Lynaugh Collection, Bryn Mawr, PA.*

nursing associations. Trevor Clay of Great Britain became the first man to serve on the board of directors; he was chosen as 1st vice president in 1989. That same year, Robert Tiffany, also of Great Britain, joined the board as member-at-large having previously served on the Professional Services Committee. More recently, Maximo Gonzalez Jurado of Spain and Cees de Ridder of the Netherlands served on the board of directors. Tesfamichael Ghebrehiwet, the first man and first African to do so, joined the ICN staff just a few years ago. The inescapable fact, however, is that men have been rare participants in the ICN, reflecting their relative scarcity in nursing in many countries of the world.

Just as men have been rare in the ICN, so women have been, and are, largely underrepresented in international organizations, both as members and leaders. This has important meaning for the ICN. Health care continues to be an arena for social change and political activism as the world grapples with how to meet the health needs of its population. A central task for the ICN, therefore, lies in its ability to respond to the private concerns and public needs of nursing as a profession while recognizing its universal role as an agent for the health and social welfare of all people.

In its role as an instrument for health and social change, the ICN must embrace foreseeable changes that may influence the continued development

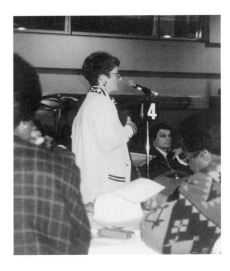

**FIGURE 6-2**
*Judith Oulton, ICN Chief Executive Officer, at the 1997 ICN Council of National Representatives, Vancouver, British Columbia, Canada. From Lynaugh Collection, Bryn Mawr, PA.*

of nurses' professionalism. For example, in 1996, Constance Holleran forecast that the globalization of nursing, privatization of health care services, advances in technology and new knowledge, and cost pressures would be major influences on nursing in the next millennium. She urged new and immediate educational improvements in computer literacy, health economics, nutrition, ethics, and an emphasis on increasing nurses' assertiveness. In 1997, the new ICN President, Kirsten Stallknecht (Denmark), urged nurses to continue to stress "humanity," reminding them that nurses "must demonstrate . . . values even when it is not always convenient for governments or others."[6]

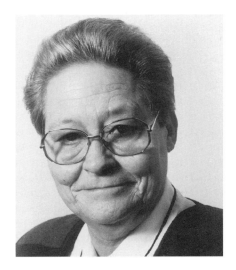

**FIGURE 6-3**
*Kirsten Stallknecht, ICN President 1997 to 2001. From ICN Collection.*

How nurses relate to their governments and nations, that is, nursing and the "state," has, as we have seen, been an issue from the founding of the ICN. Nurses' concern for the public's health, whether the threat is tuberculosis, HIV/AIDS, or the dehumanization of care through technology, is a steady theme throughout the ICN's history. Service to the nation-state in caring for the sick and injured, especially in disaster and war, is a proud element of nurses' citizenship and heritage. At the same time, nurses seek justice from the state: protection of their work from usurpation by others, fair pay, legal protection from unfair treatment, and security in carrying out their professional duties. Negotiating these areas often requires nurses to participate in the decisions that shape the political and economic contours of health care.

Indeed, as we have witnessed throughout the ICN's history, nurses have been and continue to be engaged in the politics and economics of health care as well as its practice. Particularly telling of ICN's future direction was a 1997 CNR change in the preamble of the constitution that deleted the phrase "nonpolitical," and, in its place, substituted "nonpartisan." This change aptly reflects the ICN's ongoing commitment to international involvement and political engagement.

But, as we have seen, nurses in different ICN membership countries often have different political goals. As we look ahead, the internationalization of markets may create an unknown effect on the process of reworking and redefining nursing.[7] This, coupled with generational tensions and philosophical differences among ICN member associations, may thwart or, at the very least, complicate balance between national and international interests.

The origins of the ICN are quite clear given the perspective of time, but what will be the basis for its continuation? If history offers any answer, it is that the ICN is embedded in the work of nursing and nurses. This work during the 20th century has been to care for the sick and to preserve health where possible. It seems likely that the world's societies will continue to seek out nurses to do this vital humane service, compelled by the need to sustain their economies and their people.

Nursing, as a distinct occupation, has a long history. Nursing, as a set of obligations on the part of a profession to each society it serves, is a new phenomenon of this century. As the ICN moves into the 21st century, it must continue to respond to the shifting global demands placed on professional nursing. It is the organization's enduring and vital effect on the quality, reliability, status, and socioeconomic welfare of professional nursing that is the best indicator of its future.

### ENDNOTES

1. See Barbara L. Brush and Meryn Stuart, "Unity Amidst Difference: The ICN Project and Writing International Nursing History," *Nursing History Review*, 2: 191–203.
2. See, for discussion, June Clark and Norma Lang, "The International Classification for Nursing Practice (ICNP): Nursing Outcomes," *International Nursing Review*, 44 (1997):

121–124, and, ICN, "Report of Advisory Meeting on the Development of an Informational Tool to Support Community-Based and Primary Health Care Nursing Systems," (Geneva, Switzerland: ICN, 1993).

3.  ICN Minutes, Council of National Representatives, 16–18 June 1997, pp. 15–20.

4.  ICN Minutes, Meeting of the Council of National Representatives (CNR), 16–18 June 1997, Vancouver, British Columbia, Canada. The Conselho Federal de Enfermagem of Brazil (COFEN) was admitted to membership superseding the previous ICN representative, the Brazilian Nurses Association (BNA). When COFEN applied and was voted admission, the BNA lost its voting status. This episode created a tense, sometimes bitter CNR discussion. It stood as a reminder of a series of ICN debates on which nursing organization should represent a nation dating back to the long struggle between the British Nurses' Association and the (Royal) College of Nursing in the early 1920s.

5.  ICN's interest in regulation of nursing is longstanding, but the current effort is the most sustained. See, among many reports on the project, International Council of Nurses, "Report on the Regulation of Nursing," (Margretta Styles for the Professional Services Committee; Geneva, Switzerland: ICN, 1986); Fadwa A. Affara, "Nursing Regulation—Final Report of a World Wide Project," (Geneva, Switzerland: ICN, 1992), and Fadwa A. Affara and Margretta Madden Styles, "Nursing Regulation: From Principle to Power," (The International Council of Nurses with the support of the W. K. Kellogg Foundation, ND).

6.  "An Interview with ICN's New President Kirsten Stallknecht," *ICN* 44 (1997): 131–133. Quotation is on 133.

7.  Jane Robinson, "The Internationalization of Professional Regulation," *International Nursing Review*, 42 (1995): 183–185.

# Selected Sources for This Study

Archives, International Council of Nurses, Geneva, Switzerland (ICNA).

Archives, Florence Nightingale International Foundation (FNIF), Florence Nightingale Museum, London, England.

Refugee Files, Center for the Study of the History of Nursing, University of Pennsylvania, Philadelphia, PA, USA.

Special Collections—Nursing, Mugar Library, Boston University, Boston, MA, USA.

## Selected Histories of Nursing Around the World

### GENERAL HISTORIES OF NURSING

Huda Abu-Saad, *Nursing: A World View* (St. Louis, MO and London, England: The C. V. Mosby Company, 1979).

Janice R. Ellis and Celia L. Hartley, *Nursing in Today's World: Challenges, Issues, and Trends*, 4th ed. (Philadelphia, PA: J. B. Lippincott Company, 1992).

The International Nursing Foundation of Japan, *Nursing in the World: The Facts, Needs, and Prospects*, 3rd ed. (Tokyo, Japan: Medical Friend Co., 1993).

Richard B. Splane and Verna Huffman Splane, *Chief Nursing Officer Positions in National Ministries of Health* (San Francisco, CA: University of California, 1994).

### ARGENTINA

Teresa Maria Molina, *Historia de la Enfermeria* (Editorial Intermedica, 1978)

### AUSTRALIA

Isabel 'Spark' Gill, *The Lamp Still Burns: Nursing in Victoria 1936–1981* (Maryborough, Victoria: Australian Print Group, 1989).

R. Trembath and D. Hellier, *All Care and Responsibility: A History of Nursing in Victoria, 1850–1934* (Victoria: Florence Nightingale Committee, 1987).

Barton Schultz, *A Tapestry of Service: The Evolution of Nursing in Australia, 1788–1900*, vol. I (Melbourne: Churchill Livingstone, 1991).

## BARBADOS

Eleane I. Hunte, *Barbados Registered Nurses Association Souvenir Brochure, 1936–1986* (Sunshine Publications Ltd., 1986).

## CANADA

Canadian Nurses Association, *The Leaf and the Lamp: The Seventh Decade, 1969–1980* (Canadian Nurses Association, 1981).

Canadian Nurses Association, *The Leaf and the Lamp: The Eighth Decade, 1981–1989* (Canadian Nurses Association, 1992).

## CHINA

Pao-Tien Chu, *The Developing History of the Nurses Association of the Republic of China* (The Nurses Association of the Republic of China, 1988).

## COLOMBIA

Lotty Wierner, *Remembranzas* (Self Published, 1986).

## COSTA RICA

Vilma Curling Rivera, *Charla Sobre el Colegio de Enfermeras de Costa Rica* (Documente de Archivo del Colegio, 1981).

## CUBA

Maria del Carmen Amaro, *Recuente Historico Sociedad Cubana de Enfermeria* (Unknown Publisher, 1992).

## DENMARK

Margrethe Koch, *The History of the Danish Nurses' Organization* (Copenhagen: Arnold Busk, 1944).

Esther Peterson, *From Waitress to Nurse (Episodes of the Danish Nurses' Organization)* (Copenhagen: The Danish Nurses' Organization, 1988).

Esther Peterson, *From Mission to Profession: The Fight for Government Authorization, 1899–1933* (Copenhagen: The Danish Nurses' Organization, 1989).

Esther Peterson, *Crossing the Frontiers, 1899–1940* (Copenhagen: The Danish Nurses' Organization, 1990).

## GERMANY

Ruth Elster, *Deutscher Berufsverband fur Krankenpflege: Entwicklung, Zeilsetzung, Aktivitaten, 1903–1983* (Berufsorganisation der Krankenpflegerinnen Deutschlands, 1984).

Lisotte Katscher, *Krankenpflege unde 'Drittes Reich': Der Weg der Schwesternschaft des Evangelischen Diakonievereins, 1933–1939* (Berlin: Diakonie-Verlag, no year).

Lisotte Katscher, *Krankenpflege und Zweiter Weltkrieg: Der Weg der Schwesternschaft des Evangelischen Diakonievereins Herbst 1939–Ende 1944* (Berlin: Diakonie-Verlag, no year).

Lisotte Katcher, *Krankenpflege und das Jahr 1945* (Berlin: Diakonie-Verlag, no year).

## GREAT BRITAIN

Brian Abel-Smith, *A History of Nursing Profession* (London: Heinemann, 1982).
Gerald Bowman, *The Lamp and the Book* (London: Queen Anne Press, 1967).
Susan McGann, *The Battle of the Nurses* (London: Scutari Press, 1992).
Anne Marie Rafferty, *The Politics of Nursing Knowledge* (London and New York: Routledge, 1996).

## HONDURAS

Elvia Funez de Castillo, *Sintesis Historica de la Enfermeria en Honduras* (Tegucigalpa: D. C. Mayo, 1991).

## ICELAND

Maria Petursdottir, *Hjukrunarsaga* (Self Published, 1969).

## INDIA

Suwersh K. Khauna, *The History of Nursing in India From 1947–1989* (Cape Girardeau, MO: The Nursing Society of India, Inc., 1991).
Ranjana Raghavachari, *Conflicts and Adjustments: Indian Nurses in an Urban Milieu* (UBS Publishers Distributors LTD Delhi: Academic Foundation, 1990).
Alice Wilkenson, *A Brief History of Nursing in India and Pakistan* (The Trained Nurses' Association of India, 1958).

## IRELAND

Pauline Scanlon, *The Irish Nurse: A Study of Nursing in Ireland: History and Education, 1718–1981* (Leitrim, Ireland: Drumlin Publications Ltd., 1991).

## LIBERIA

J. Birney Dibble, *Outlaw for God: The Esther Bacon Story* (Hanover, MA: The Christopher Publishing House, 1992).

## NEPAL

Sumitra Bantawa and Tara Thladhar, *Nursing Souvenir* (Nepal: Nursing Association of Nepal, 1991).

## NEW ZEALAND

Helen Campbell, *Mary Lambie: A Biography* (Wellington, New Zealand: The New Zealand Nursing Education and Research Foundation, 1976).
Margaret Gibson Smith and Yvonne Shadbolt, *Objects and Outcomes: The New Zealand Nurses' Association, 1909–1983* (Wellington: New Zealand Nurses' Association, Inc., 1984).

NICARAGUA

Soledad Galeano Plazaola, *La Enfermeria en Nicaragua* (Publicanciones Nicaraguenses S. A., 1974).

NORWAY

Kari Melby, *Kall og Kamp: Norsk Sykepleier Forbunds Historie* (Oslo, Norway: Norsk Sykepleier Forbund, 1990).
Nete Balslev Wingender, *The Northern Nurses' Federation, 1920–1995* (Oslo, Norway: Northern Nurses' Federation, 1995).
Ingrid Wyller, *Norsk Sykepleier Forbund, 1912–1962* (Oslo, Norway: Norsk Sykepleier Forbund, 1962).

PANAMA

Junta Directiva de Esa Epoca, *Memoria de Anep-Bodas de Oro* (Lic. Gladis de Lam, 1975).

PHILIPPINES

Anastacia Giron-Tupas, *History of Nursing in the Philippines* (Manila: Anastacia Giron-Tupas, 1958).

POLAND

Irena Wronska, *Polskie Peilegniarstwo, 1921–1939* (Norbertium, 1991).

SOUTH AFRICA

Shula Marks, *Divided Sisterhood—Race, Class and Gender in the South African Nursing Profession* (New York: St. Martin's Press, 1994).

SWEDEN

Eva Bohm, *Okand-Godkand-Legitimerad* (Stockholm: Sjukskoterskeforbundet, 1961).
Gerd Zetterstrom, *Systerskap i Forandring* (Stockholm: Sjukskoterskeforbundet, 1985).

THAILAND

Sooluk Muchoosub (ed.), *Sixty Years Anniversary of the Nurses' Association of Thailand* (Siam Publishing Company, 1987).

UNITED STATES

Darlene Clark Hine, *Black Women in White—Racial Conflict and Cooperation in the Nursing Profession, 1890–1950* (Bloomington and Indianapolis: Indiana University Press, 1989).
Phillip A. Kalisch and Beatrice J. Kalisch, *The Advance of American Nursing* (Boston and Toronto: Little, Brown and Company, 1986).
Joan E. Lynaugh and Barbara L. Brush, *American Nursing—From Hospitals to Health Systems* (Oxford and Cambridge, MA: Blackwell Publishers, 1996).
Susan Reverby, *Ordered to Care—The Dilemma of American Nursing, 1850–1945* (Cambridge, London, and New York: Cambridge University Press, 1987).

# APPENDIX II

# The Presidents of ICN and Their Watchwords

| Year | President | Watchword |
|------|-----------|-----------|
| 1901 | Ethel Bedford Fenwick | Work |
| 1904 | Susan McGahey | Courage |
| 1909 | Agnes Karll | Life |
| 1912 | Annie Goodrich | Aspiration |
| 1915 | Henny Tscherning | —— |
| 1922 | Sophie Mannerheim | —— |
| 1925 | Nina Gage | Peace |
| 1929 | Leonie Chaptal | Service |
| 1933 | Alicia Lloyd Still | Concordia |
| 1937 | Effie Taylor | Loyalty |
| 1947 | Gerda Hojer | Faith |
| 1953 | Marie Bihet | Responsibility |
| 1957 | Agnes Ohlson | Wisdom |
| 1961 | Alice Clamageran | Enquiry |
| 1965 | Alice Girard | Tenacity |
| 1969 | Margrethe Kruse | Unity |
| 1973 | Dorothy Cornelius | Flexibility |
| 1977 | Olive Anstrey | Accountability |
| 1981 | Eunice Muringo Kiereini | —— |
| 1985 | Nelly Garzon | Freedom |
| 1989 | Mo-Im Kim | Justice |
| 1993 | Margretta Nadden Styles | Love |
| 1997 | Kirsten Stallknecht | Humanity |

# APPENDIX III

## Executives of the International Council of Nurses

Christiane Reimann — Secretary, then Executive Secretary 1992–1933

Anna Schwarzenberg — Executive Secretary 1934–1947

Daisy Bridges — Executive, then General Secretary 1948–1961

Helen Nussbaum — General Secretary 1961–1967

Sheila Quinn — Executive Director 1968–1970

Adele Herwitz — Executive Director 1970–1977

Barbara Fawkes — Executive Director 1977–1978

Winifred Logan — Executive Director 1978–1980

Constance Holleran — Executive Director 1981–1996

Judith Oulton — Chief Executive Officer 1996–present

# INDEX

References with "f" denote figures

## A

acquired immunodeficiency syndrome, 171, 173, 181
Africa, nursing in, 130–131
AIDS. *See* acquired immunodeficiency syndrome
American Medical Association, 183
American Nurses Association, 183
American Society of Superintendents of Training Schools for Nurses, 40–41
ANA. *See* American Nurses Association
Anstey, Olive E., 163–164
Anthony, Susan B., 11
antislavery movement, 8
apartheid, 137–138, 151–153
ASSTSN. *See* American Society of Superintendents of Training Schools for Nurses

## B

*Basic Principles of Nursing Care*, 135
Berlin Congress (1904) meeting, 24, 30–32
Bihet, Marie, 127–128
British College of Nursing
  affiliation with International Council of Nurses, 81–82
  description of, 82
British Nurses Association, 12–13
Buffalo Congress (1901) meeting, 19–24

## C

Chaptal, Leonie Marie, 93–94
China
  American Rockefeller Foundation involvement in, 87
  civil war in, 88–89
  customs regarding women, 87
  International Council of Nurses participation in, 86–88, 126
  Nurses' Association of, 132
  nursing in, 86–88, 119, 132
  political views, 86–87
Chinese Nurses' Association, 174–175
Clamageran, Alice, 138f, 138–140
CNA. *See* Chinese Nurses' Association
colonialism, 101–104, 130
Copenhagen Congress (1922) meeting, 63–64, 77
Cornelius, Dorothy, 156, 157f, 160, 164

## D

diagnosis-related groups, 183
Dock, Lavinia, 2f, 3, 16, 18, 32–33, 42, 57–58, 120–121
DRG. *See* diagnosis-related groups

## E

ECNE. *See* European Council for Nursing Education
education, of nurses, 13, 31, 50, 64, 90–91, 158
European Council for Nursing Education, 81
Exchange of Nurses Committee, 124

## F

female genital mutilation, 165–166, 186
Fenwick, Ethel Gordon, 1
  death of, 120
  illustration of, 2f
  in International Council of Nurses, 16–17, 19–20, 31, 40

## DATE DUE

NOV 0 1 2011